Evolving Concepts in Insulin Resistance

Edited by Marco Infante

Published in London, United Kingdom

Evolving Concepts in Insulin Resistance
http://dx.doi.org/10.5772/intechopen.98058
Edited by Marco Infante

Contributors
Patricio H. Contreras, Noah Moruzzi, Francesca Lazzeri-Barcelo, Preet Mohinder Singh Bedi, Nikhita Ghai, Atamjit Singh, Asish K. Saha, Barry Sears, Mustafa Öztop, Marco Infante, Martina Leoni, Nathalia Padilla, Andrea Fabbri, David Della-Morte, Camillo Ricordi

First published in London, United Kingdom, 2022 by IntechOpen
IntechOpen is the global imprint of INTECHOPEN LIMITED, registered in England and Wales, registration number: 11086078, 5 Princes Gate Court, London, SW7 2QJ, United Kingdom

British Library Cataloguing-in-Publication Data
A catalogue record for this book is available from the British Library

Additional hard and PDF copies can be obtained from orders@intechopen.com

Evolving Concepts in Insulin Resistance
Edited by Marco Infante
p. cm.
Print ISBN 978-1-80355-501-0
Online ISBN 978-1-80355-502-7
eBook (PDF) ISBN 978-1-80355-503-4

Meet the editor

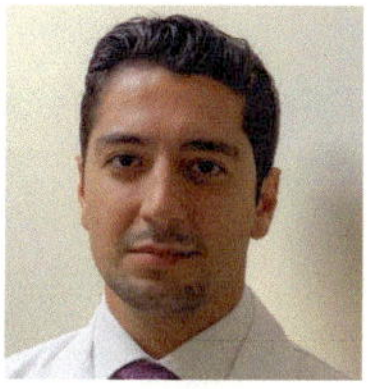

Marco Infante serves as an Adjunct Professor of Endocrinology and Adjunct Professor of Applied Nutrition in Internal Medicine at Saint Camillus International University of Health Sciences (Rome, Italy). He serves as Research Scholar at the Diabetes Research Institute (DRI), University of Miami Miller School of Medicine (USA). He received the designation as a Fellow of the American College of Nutrition (FACN) by virtue of his research activity in the field of "Immunomodulatory Nutrition". He is a member of several international scientific organizations, including the *Diabetes Research Institute Federation*. Dr. Infante also serves as the Academic Editor of the *Journal of Diabetes Research*. He authored numerous publications in international peer-reviewed journals and gave lectures at international diabetes meetings.

Contents

Preface

Over the last decades, the growing prevalence of insulin resistance has dramatically contributed to the global epidemic of metabolic syndrome, obesity, type 2 diabetes mellitus, and cardiovascular disease. Therefore, there is an unmet need for novel nutritional and pharmacological strategies aimed to prevent or treat insulin resistance and its related comorbidities. In this book, internationally renowned experts present the latest insights into the pathophysiology and clinical consequences of insulin resistance in different settings, describing novel diagnostic biomarkers and molecular targets of this condition. I trust that researchers and clinicians will find this text informative and useful to expand their knowledge of the molecular mechanisms underlying insulin resistance, prompting the future clinical translation of the latest scientific discoveries in the field. Finally, I wish to express my sincere thanks to IntechOpen and the authors who contributed to this book.

Marco Infante, MD, FACN
Adjunct Professor of Endocrinology,
Faculty of Medicine and Surgery,
UniCamillus, Saint Camillus International University of Health Sciences,
Rome, Italy

Adjunct Professor of Applied Nutrition in Internal Medicine,
Master Degree Course in Human Nutrition Sciences,
UniCamillus, Saint Camillus International University of Health Sciences,
Rome, Italy

Research Scholar,
Diabetes Research Institute (DRI) and Cell Transplant Center,
University of Miami Miller School of Medicine,
Miami, FL, USA

Diabetes Research Institute Federation (DRIF),
Department of Systems Medicine,
University of Rome Tor Vergata,
Rome, Italy

Fellow of the American College of Nutrition

Foreword

Evolving Concepts in Insulin Resistance provides an updated, authoritative, and comprehensive text that rigorously and elegantly describes novel molecular mechanisms accounting for the development of insulin resistance. Readers will pleasantly get carried away through the stages of the insulin journey in the human body, gaining new insights into defects in insulin signaling and novel molecular targets of insulin resistance.

Camillo Ricordi, MD, FNAI
Stacy Joy Goodman Professor of Surgery and Chief,
Division of Cellular Transplantation,

Distinguished Professor of Medicine,

Professor of Biomedical Engineering, Microbiology and Immunology,

Director,
Diabetes Research Institute (DRI) and Cell Transplant Center,
University of Miami Miller School of Medicine,
Miami, FL, USA

Fellow of the National Academy of Inventors,
USA

Member of the Italian Supreme Council of Health

Chapter 1

The Insulin Journey in the Human Body

Marco Infante

Abstract

Insulin represents the paramount anabolic hormone and the master regulator of glucose, lipid, and protein metabolism. This chapter describes the sequential stages of the physiologic journey of insulin in the human body, from its synthesis/secretion to its action in peripheral tissues and, ultimately, to its clearance and degradation. These stages include i) insulin synthesis and release from pancreatic beta cells; ii) insulin first-pass metabolism and partial clearance in the liver; iii) insulin action on the vasculature and exit from the capillary beds; iv) insulin action in peripheral and central target tissues (skeletal muscle, adipose tissue, liver, and central nervous system); and v) final insulin degradation in the kidney. Each of these stages is regulated by complex intracellular mechanisms that take place in different tissues and allow for the anabolic actions of insulin. Understanding the abovementioned stages is pivotal to comprehending the clinical consequences of impaired insulin secretion and action, as defects in one or more of these stages can be associated with the development of insulin resistance, metabolic syndrome, and type 2 diabetes mellitus. Additionally, a thorough knowledge of the insulin bodily journey can assist clinicians in therapeutic decision-making for diabetic patients on exogenous insulin therapy in different clinical settings.

Keywords: insulin synthesis, insulin secretion, insulin action, insulin metabolism, beta cell, liver, vasculature, skeletal muscle, adipose tissue, brain, kidney, glucose metabolism

1. Introduction

The year 2021 marked the 100th anniversary of the discovery of insulin, which was first isolated from a dog's pancreas by Frederick Grant Banting and Charles Herbert Best under the directorship of John James Rickard Macleod at the University of Toronto in 1921. Insulin purification was then made possible by James Collip. The Nobel Prize in Physiology or Medicine 1923 was awarded jointly to Frederick Grant Banting and John James Rickard Macleod for the discovery of insulin. This groundbreaking discovery has since saved and improved the lives of millions of people with diabetes worldwide [1].

This chapter aims to describe in detail the sequential stages of the physiologic journey of insulin in the human body, from its synthesis and secretion to its action in central and peripheral target tissues and, ultimately, to its clearance and degradation. Specifically, the chapter will focus on five essential stages of the insulin bodily journey, namely: i) insulin biosynthesis and release from pancreatic beta cells; ii) insulin first-pass metabolism and partial clearance in the liver; iii) insulin action on the vasculature and exit from the capillary beds; iv) insulin action in skeletal muscle, adipose tissue, liver, and central nervous system (CNS); v) final insulin degradation in the kidney [2]. Understanding such stages is clinically relevant, as defects in one or more of them can be associated with insulin resistance [2–5]. In turn, insulin resistance is often associated with a cluster of cardiometabolic conditions (e.g., type 2 diabetes mellitus, obesity, atherosclerosis, and cardiovascular disease) that are collectively known as the metabolic syndrome (a.k.a. "insulin resistance syndrome") and can result in high cardiovascular morbidity and mortality rates [6, 7]. Additionally, a thorough knowledge of the insulin bodily journey can assist clinicians in therapeutic decision-making for diabetic patients on exogenous insulin therapy in different clinical settings.

2. Insulin biosynthesis and release from pancreatic beta cells

Human insulin is a 51-amino acid peptide hormone synthesized and secreted by the pancreatic beta cells present within the islets of Langerhans. It consists of two polypeptide chains (A chain and B chain) linked together by two disulfide bonds (with an additional disulfide present within the A chain). The A chain consists of 21 amino acids, whereas the B chain consists of 30 amino acids. Insulin represents the paramount anabolic hormone promoting dietary carbon source deposition, with its major action sites being represented by the liver, skeletal muscle, and adipose tissue [2]. Production and secretion of insulin from pancreatic beta cells are crucial to maintaining normoglycemia. In humans, the insulin gene (INS) is located on chromosome 11. Its transcription is regulated by transcription factors (e.g., Pdx-1, NeuroD1, MafA) in response to increased circulating glucose levels [8]. Changes in glucose concentrations influence these beta-cell transcription factors at multiple levels, leading to parallel changes in their subcellular localization, expression levels, DNA-binding activity, transactivation capacity, and interaction with other proteins [8]. Once secreted, insulin exerts its functions by binding the insulin receptor (IR) expressed on target tissues. IR is a member of the ligand-activated receptor and tyrosine kinase family of transmembrane signaling proteins. The IR is a dimer of heterodimers that comprises two α-chains and two β-chains [9]. The human IR (hINSR) gene spans a region of greater than 120,000 base pairs (bp) on the short arm of chromosome 19 [10]. The Insulin Receptor Substrate (IRS) proteins represent a family of cytoplasmic adaptor proteins that transmit signals from the insulin and insulin-like growth factor 1 (IGF-1) receptors to evoke a cellular response [11].

In pancreatic beta cells, insulin is initially translated as preproinsulin, which is subsequently processed to proinsulin in the rough endoplasmic reticulum (RER) after the cleavage of its N-terminal signal peptide mediated by a signal peptidase. C-peptide (a.k.a. the connecting peptide) is a short 31-amino-acid peptide that connects insulin's A-chain to its B-chain in the proinsulin molecule. In the RER, proinsulin undergoes rapid folding and disulfide bond formation. During this stage, the placement of C-peptide promotes the proper formation of disulfide bonds within and between the A and B peptide chains. After transit to the Golgi complex, proinsulin is sorted into immature secretory granules, where it is processed by prohormone convertases (PCSK1 and PCSK2) that act by cleaving the C-peptide. C-peptide is subsequently released into the bloodstream as a by-product of proinsulin proteolysis. Then, carboxypeptidase E (CPE) removes C-terminal basic amino acids from the resulting peptide chains, leading to the formation of mature insulin, a peptide hormone containing 51 amino acids distributed among the A and B chains of 21 and 30 amino acids, respectively. A and B chains are linked by two disulfide bonds, while another disulfide bond is formed within the A chain (**Figure 1**) [2, 12]. The zinc (Zn^{2+}) cation co-crystallizes with insulin to form a hexameric crystal in the mature secretory granules. The zinc transporter 8 (ZnT8) or related zinc transporters have been suggested to mediate the transport of the insulin hexamer into the secretory granules [13]. Insulin granules dock with the plasma membrane through the coordinated interaction and recruitment of exocytic SNARE (soluble N-ethylmaleimide-sensitive-factor attachment protein receptor) proteins [14]. Indeed, loss or altered activity of key SNARE proteins results in impaired insulin secretion [15].

Insulin synthesis is generally rapid (< 2 hours) and highly efficient, as only 1–2% of the protein remains as proinsulin within mature secretory granules. Hyperproinsulinemia indicates a pathological state arising from inefficient proinsulin processing within the beta-cell secretory granules and/or from premature release of proinsulin [16]. Indeed, the circulating proinsulin-to-C-peptide ratio (PI:C ratio) and proinsulin-to-insulin ratio (PIR) can be used as biomarkers of beta-cell endoplasmic reticulum dysfunction and inefficient proinsulin processing [17–19]. On the other hand, C-peptide is routinely used as a surrogate marker of endogenous insulin secretion due to the following reasons: C-peptide is secreted from pancreatic beta cells at an equimolar ratio to endogenous insulin, has negligible hepatic clearance, and is excreted at a more constant rate over a longer time compared to insulin, and its concentrations are not influenced by therapeutically administered exogenous insulin [20].

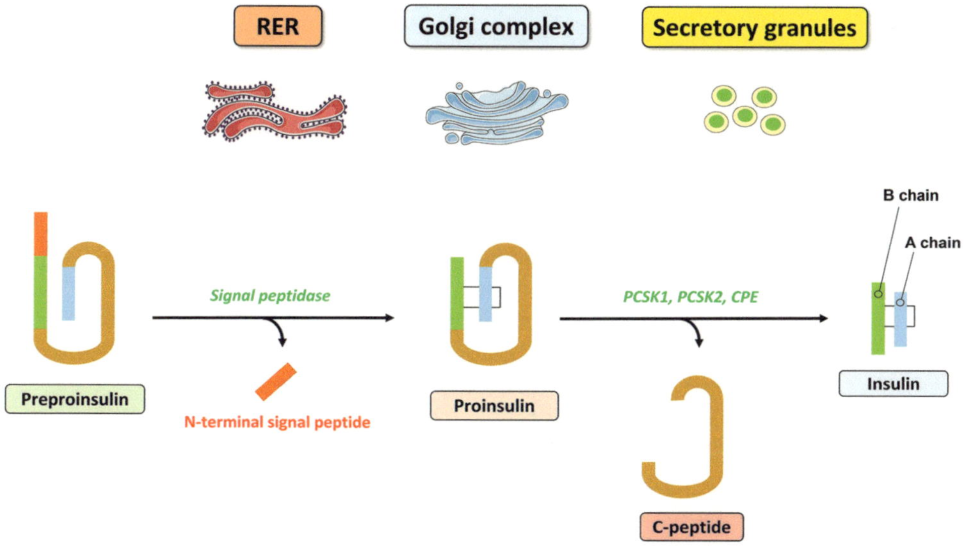

Figure 1.
Physiologic stages of proinsulin processing in insulin-secreting pancreatic beta cells. Abbreviations: CPE, carboxypeptidase E; PCSK1, Proprotein convertase Subtilisin/Kexin type 1; PCSK2, Proprotein convertase Subtilisin/Kexin type 2; RER, rough endoplasmic reticulum. The figure was partly created with images adapted from Servier Medical Art licensed under a creative commons attribution 3.0 Unported license (https://smart.servier.com/).

2.1 Biphasic insulin secretion

Glucose-stimulated insulin secretion (GSIS) *in vitro* consists of a transient first phase followed by a more sustained second phase. Shortly after the increase in glucose concentration following a meal, there is a transient stimulation of insulin secretion referred to as "first phase secretion." This phase is then followed by a gradually developing secondary stimulation referred to as "second phase secretion" [21]. This biphasic insulin secretion reflects exocytosis of two distinct functional subsets of secretory granules in different pools [21]. Most granules (> 95%) belong to the reserve pool and are not available for release until they are physically translocated or chemically modified. The other subset of granules is referred to as the "readily releasable pool (RRP)" and contains less than 5% of the total granule number. Secretory granules proceed from the reserve pool into the RRP through a process called "mobilization," which involves one or several ATP-dependent reactions [21, 22]. During the mobilization toward the cell periphery, granules must cross a cortical actin network to reach the plasma membrane. The rapid first phase of insulin secretion lasts up to 10 minutes and results from the fusion of the RRP granules with the plasma membrane. The RRP granules are already located at the membrane under basal conditions; these granules discharge their cargo in response to nutrient and non-nutrient secretagogues. The first phase of insulin secretion is then followed by a second phase associated with actin reorganization (to allow the recruitment of insulin secretory granules to the plasma membrane) and reaches a plateau at 2–3 hours [23]. Unlike the first phase, the second phase of insulin secretion can be evoked by nutrients and fuel secretagogues (like glucose) only and involves the mobilization of intracellular granules to t-SNARE sites at the plasma membrane to allow the distal docking and fusion steps of insulin exocytosis [24]. Thus, the actin cytoskeleton acts as a physical barrier to insulin secretion [24]. Conversely, the first phase secretion can also be elicited by non-metabolizable stimuli, suggesting that the second phase of insulin secretion represents an energy-dependent process. In type 2 diabetes mellitus (T2DM), there are alterations in the insulin release pattern that selectively involve the first phase of insulin secretion. This selective loss of the first phase insulin secretion can be the earliest detectable defect of beta-cell function after years of compensation for antecedent insulin resistance in subjects predisposed to develop T2DM. However, early abnormalities in the second phase of insulin secretion have also been described [21, 23].

2.2 Glucose sensing in pancreatic beta cells and insulin granule exocytosis

All the steps leading to the arrival, priming, docking, and fusion of secretory granules are regulated by a series of physiologic signals initiated by glucose, which represents the paramount metabolic signal evoking insulin secretion.

In humans, glucose enters the beta cell through glucose transporter type 1 (GLUT1) expressed on the cell membrane [25]. Afterward, the enzyme glucokinase (GK)—an isoform of hexokinase—rapidly phosphorylates glucose, leading to production of glucose-6-phosphate (G6P), which fuels the mitochondrial tricarboxylic acid (TCA) cycle via glycolysis and pyruvate generation. The completion of the TCA cycle leads to generation of ATP (adenosine triphosphate) from ADP (adenosine diphosphate) by ATP synthase, resulting in increases in the cytosolic ATP/ADP ratio. In turn, the increases in the cytosolic ATP/ADP ratio regulate cell membrane potential through inhibition and closure of ATP-sensitive K^+ (K_{ATP}) channels, thus generating cell membrane depolarization (conversion of chemical to electrical signaling). When a certain threshold potential is exceeded (−55 mV to −50 mV), voltage-dependent Na^+ and Ca^{2+} channels are activated and cause repetitive action potential spiking. The Ca^{2+} influx via voltage-gated Ca^{2+} channels results in the elevation of intracellular Ca^{2+} concentration, which subsequently triggers the fusion of the insulin granule bilayer with the plasma membrane (insulin granule exocytosis) and the release of insulin from the beta cell [26].

Although insulin is secreted primarily in response to glucose, additional nutrients and metabolic factors can amplify the glucose-induced insulin secretion, such as the gut-derived hormones called incretins (glucagon-like peptide-1 and glucose-dependent insulinotropic polypeptide), free fatty acids (FFAs), and amino acids [27]. Beta cells release insulin directly into the interstitial space of the pancreas, which is surrounded by a fenestrated endothelium that permits insulin to find its way into the portal circulation readily and to undergo the first-pass metabolism in the liver subsequently.

Beta cells' electrical and Ca^{2+} responses within a pancreatic islet are synchronized thanks to gap junctions and paracrine and autocrine signals (e.g., ATP) [28–30]. The communication between beta cells within pancreatic islets contributes to the oscillations in insulin secretion, which occurs with a periodicity of 5–10 minutes in healthy individuals [31]. Yet, it is still unclear how several individual islets within the human pancreas (approximately one million) communicate and synchronize their insulin secretory oscillations to allow a pulsatile insulin release from the whole pancreas [2]. In this regard, it has been suggested that an intrapancreatic neural network may coordinate activity among different islet populations [2, 32].

3. First-pass hepatic insulin clearance and insulin action in the liver

Although pancreatic beta cells secrete insulin, the liver acts as a gatekeeper that regulates the amount of insulin allowed to reach the systemic circulation for action on target peripheral tissues through a process called "first-pass insulin clearance." Therefore, the liver is the first organ that insulin encounters along its journey in the human body. It acts as a buffer to prevent peripheral hyperinsulinemia and subsequent insulin resistance in skeletal muscle and adipose tissue [6, 33]. The hepatic portal vein, which is the main vessel of the portal venous system, drains the blood from the gastrointestinal tract, gallbladder, pancreas, and spleen to the liver. As such, the portal vein also delivers insulin from the pancreas to the liver in discrete pulses occurring approximately every 5 minutes [34]. The magnitude of these insulin pulses varies between 0.5 and 1 nmol/L in the fasting state and ~5 nmol/L after a meal [34, 35]. Enhanced insulin release in response to hyperglycemia is achieved by amplifying these high-frequency pulses [34]. The pulsatile insulin delivery through the portal vein to the liver regulates both hepatic insulin action and hepatic insulin extraction [36, 37].

Insulin reaches the liver through the portal vein at concentrations up to 10-fold higher than the insulin concentrations in the systemic circulation, thus creating a "portal-systemic gradient" mainly maintained by the significant hepatic insulin degradation [38]. Hence, the liver is exposed to substantially higher insulin concentrations than other insulin-responsive tissues such as skeletal muscle and adipose tissue.

Hepatocytes represent the cellular site where insulin clearance takes place. After its release into the portal circulation, insulin reaches the capillaries of the hepatic sinusoids, which, unlike other blood vessels, lack a basement membrane and are lined only by fenestrated (porous) endothelial cells [39]. The unique structure of hepatic sinusoids allows the exchange of contents between the blood and the surrounding hepatocytes. Thus, insulin easily diffuses from the portal circulation into the perisinusoidal space (the space between the sinusoids and the hepatocytes) and directly interacts with the hepatocyte surface. Receptor-mediated insulin uptake followed by insulin degradation in hepatocytes represents the underlying mechanism of hepatic insulin clearance [40]. Insulin binds the IR located on the microvilli of the hepatocyte membrane. The IR-insulin complex (receptor-ligand complex) is then internalized through clathrin-mediated endocytosis [41–43]. The subsequent loss of IR on the hepatocyte surface is followed by rapid recycling and reinsertion of intact and unbound IRs in the plasma membrane [44]. Michael *et al.* [45] showed that liver-specific insulin receptor knockout (LIRKO) mice exhibit dramatic insulin resistance due to alterations in the IR-mediated insulin endocytosis and degradation, which resulted in marked hyperinsulinemia due to a combination of increased insulin secretion and decreased insulin clearance. These findings support the importance of physiologic hepatic insulin signaling in regulating glucose homeostasis and maintaining normal liver function.

Hepatocytes express high levels of the enzyme CEACAM1 (carcinoembryonic antigen-related cell adhesion molecule 1), a transmembrane glycoprotein phosphorylated by the IR and allowing the formation of an insulin-IR-CEACAM1 complex [46]. This complex upregulates the IR-mediated insulin endocytosis and degradation. The importance of CEACAM1 in hepatic insulin clearance has been demonstrated by animal studies showing that defects in insulin-stimulated hepatic CEACAM1 phosphorylation led to severe hyperinsulinemia and consequential insulin resistance, impaired glucose tolerance, and hyperglycemia [47]. The insulin degradation process begins upon insulin binding to the hepatocyte plasma membrane, where insulin is partly degraded by the extracellular insulin-degrading enzyme (IDE) [48]. The remaining insulin is degraded after internalization into the hepatocyte by IDE in endosomes and through proteolysis in lysosomes [2].

The half-life of insulin in the portal circulation is ~3–5 minutes [49]. Under physiologic conditions, up to 80% (usually 50%) of secreted insulin is degraded during its first-pass hepatic clearance [50]. Thus, the insulin concentration in the systemic circulation is about one-third that in the portal circulation (3:1 ratio of hepatic to peripheral insulin levels). The remaining undegraded insulin exits the liver through the hepatic veins and reaches the heart through the inferior vena cava. The heart then pumps insulin into the systemic (arterial) circulation toward the target tissues (skeletal muscle, adipose tissue, liver, and brain), where insulin exerts its actions. Approximately 25% of undegraded insulin returns to the liver (specifically, to the hepatic sinusoids) via the hepatic artery and undergoes a second round of insulin degradation in the hepatocytes ("second-pass hepatic insulin clearance") [2].

Hepatic insulin degradation represents a physiologic mechanism modulating the amount of insulin that reaches the systemic circulation according to the metabolic demands and the insulin concentration that is required in the periphery. Under pathological conditions characterized by insulin resistance (e.g., obesity), there is a decreased hepatic insulin clearance rate that compensates for reduced peripheral insulin sensitivity and contributes (together with an increased insulin secretion rate) to the compensatory hyperinsulinemia of insulin-resistant individuals [51]. In this regard, Lee *et al.* showed that CEACAM1 expression is decreased in the hepatocytes of diabetic and nondiabetic patients with severe obesity and fatty liver disease, both of which are conditions commonly associated with insulin resistance [52].

3.1 Insulin action in the liver

Besides being involved in insulin degradation, the liver represents a major target tissue where insulin acts through the phosphoinositide 3-kinase (PI3K)/Akt pathway, which is a key signaling pathway mediating the insulin effects on anabolic metabolism in all organisms [3, 53]. Notably, insulin regulates hepatic glucose output by promoting glycolysis and glycogen synthesis (via activation of glycogen synthase) and by suppressing gluconeogenesis (*de novo* glucose production) and glycogenolysis (glycogen breakdown) [54]. This mechanism of action permits the hepatic storage of glucose as glycogen so that the hepatic glucose output prevails in the interprandial periods (when insulin action ceases) and/or upon stimulation by counterregulatory hormones (predominantly glucagon) that promote hepatic glycogenolysis and gluconeogenesis [55].

Glycogen synthesis (a.k.a. glycogenesis) and glycogenolysis are reciprocal pathways regulated by the balance between circulating insulin and glucagon concentrations under fed and fasting conditions, respectively [6]. Glucose production by the liver is finely regulated by insulin and counterregulatory hormones (e.g., glucagon), neural mechanisms, and nutrient supply. After glucose ingestion, insulin is released from the pancreatic beta cells into the portal circulation. It potently and rapidly inhibits hepatic glucose production (HPG) by directly suppressing glycogenolysis via the PI3K/Akt pathway, inhibiting the glycogen phosphorylase [6]. At this stage, insulin also promotes hepatic glucose uptake and glucose storage as glycogen by activating the enzyme glycogen synthase phosphatase, which catalyzes the dephosphorylation and subsequent activation of glycogen synthase [6, 56]. Moreover, insulin released from pancreatic beta cells after a meal suppresses HPG through its ability to inhibit the pancreatic alpha cell secretion of glucagon [57], a well-known counterregulatory hormone that stimulates hepatic gluconeogenesis [58].

Hepatic gluconeogenesis consists of the synthesis of glucose from non-carbohydrate precursors (such as lactate, pyruvate, glycerol, propionate, and alanine). It contributes to approximately 50% of all HGP following overnight fasting [6]. Although the liver is the major site of gluconeogenesis, a smaller contribution to this process is also provided by the kidney, small intestine, skeletal muscle, and brain [59–62].

In the fed state, insulin inhibits hepatic gluconeogenesis primarily via direct mechanisms by acting as a potent negative regulator of different gluconeogenic enzymes in hepatocytes—such as glucose 6-phosphatase (G6Pase) and phosphoenolpyruvate carboxykinase (PEPCK)—after its release into the portal circulation [6, 63–65]. However, insulin-mediated inhibition of hepatic gluconeogenesis also occurs through indirect mechanisms, namely via the insulin-mediated suppression of lipolysis, which results in decreased FFA availability and reduced hepatic acetyl-coenzyme A (acetyl-CoA) levels. Yet, this indirect pathway becomes relevant mainly when insulin is administered peripherally, and the physiologic (positive) portal-systemic blood insulin gradient is disrupted [6].

Under fasting conditions, glucagon inhibits the activity of the enzyme pyruvate kinase (PK), thus promoting the utilization of phosphoenolpyruvate for gluconeogenesis. In the fed state, insulin counteracts this process, favoring the uptake and oxidation of glucose in the liver [6, 66].

In the liver, insulin also controls lipid homeostasis by stimulating *de novo* lipogenesis and by regulating hepatic triacylglycerol (TAG) secretion via very-low-density lipoprotein (VLDL)-TAG export. This is in line with insulin acting as an anabolic hormone that promotes energy storage in both liver and adipose tissue. Specifically, insulin regulates VLDL production in the liver by targeting apolipoprotein B (apoB) for degradation and reducing apoB synthesis [67]. In the postprandial period, the increase in portal insulin concentrations reduces hepatic VLDL output and allows for temporary triglyceride storage for future secretion. Indeed, insulin induction of hepatic *de novo* lipogenesis favors triglyceride synthesis and occurs independently of insulin effects on apoB. Under conditions of insulin resistance, there is a higher apoB availability, which results in hepatic VLDL hypersecretion (coupled with stimulation of hepatic *de novo* lipogenesis). In turn, the hepatic VLDL hypersecretion results in the packaging of excess triglycerides into larger-sized VLDL particles (termed VLDL1) and more numerous VLDL particles, thus inducing hypertriglyceridemia [68]. Indeed, enhanced secretion of VLDL-TAG and hypertriglyceridemia are hallmarks of insulin-resistant conditions, such as obesity or non-alcoholic fatty liver disease (NAFLD) [53].

4. Insulin action in the vasculature

In systemic circulation, insulin starts to exert its hemodynamic effects on the vessels by promoting vasodilation and increasing blood flow to allow its own delivery to the peripheral tissues. In the macrovasculature, insulin binds the IR expressed on the endothelial cells and leads to the phosphorylation of the insulin receptor substrate 2 (IRS-2), which, in turn, results in the activation of class I PI3K that is linked downstream to the Akt/PKB (protein kinase B) signaling pathway. The downstream activation of Akt causes phosphorylation and activation of endothelial nitric oxide synthase (eNOS), which, in turn, catalyzes the synthesis of nitric oxide (NO) from L-arginine [69]. Subsequently, NO rapidly and freely diffuses to the adjacent outer layer of vascular smooth muscle cells (VSMCs), where it activates the intracellular enzyme guanylate cyclase that converts guanosine triphosphate (GTP) to cyclic guanosine monophosphate (cGMP). The increase in intracellular cGMP concentration results in the activation of protein kinase G (PKG), which, in turn, causes reductions in intracellular Ca^{2+} concentration and subsequent relaxation of vascular smooth muscle and vasodilation *via* activation of the myosin light-chain phosphatase [70]. Insulin action in target tissues is temporally linked to the insulin's vascular effects. For example, insulin acts on the vasculature to enhance its own delivery to skeletal muscle by inducing the relaxation of resistance vessels to increase blood flow and by promoting the relaxation of precapillary arterioles to increase the microvascular exchange surface perfused within the skeletal muscle (microvascular recruitment) [71]. Thus, insulin rapidly recruits skeletal muscle capillaries by a NO-dependent action, and the increase in capillary recruitment represents an early insulin effect promoting glucose uptake by the perfused myocytes [72]. Indeed, microvascular recruitment precedes both the activation of insulin signaling pathways and the increases in glucose disposal in skeletal muscle [72]. Under resting conditions, only 30–50% of muscle capillaries are perfused, and this proportion increases 2- to 3-fold in response to exercise and insulin action [6, 73]. During insulin resistance and in the presence of diabetes, obesity, and/or use of nitric oxide synthase inhibitors, vasoactive effects of insulin (including microvascular recruitment) can be impaired [71, 74–76].

When insulin reaches the capillaries of its target tissues (skeletal muscle and adipose tissue), it must pass through the capillary's continuous endothelial lining to access the interstitial space and the parenchymal cells (myocytes and adipocytes). As capillaries are composed of a single layer of endothelial cells with interendothelial junctions, two possible routes have been proposed to explain the mechanism of insulin egress from the microvascular capillary endothelium toward the interstitial space and the parenchyma tissues (skeletal muscle and adipose tissue). In particular, insulin may cross the capillary endothelia via a transcellular route (through individual endothelial cells via receptor-mediated endocytosis and/or via fluid-phase endocytosis) or via a paracellular route (between adjacent endothelial cells) [2, 77].

It is worth noting that NO acts as a potent vasodilator and antiatherogenic molecule. NO synthesis is stimulated by insulin in VSMCs [78]. Thus, insulin exerts cardioprotective effects, whereas insulin resistance alters the NO synthesis causing accelerated atherosclerosis, coronary artery disease, and hypertension (all conditions frequently associated with obesity and/or T2DM). In addition, hyperinsulinemia secondary to insulin resistance leads to stimulation of the mitogen-activated protein kinase (MAPK) pathway, which results in enhanced VSMC growth and proliferation, inflammation, and atherosclerosis [79]. This occurs because MAPK can be activated either by insulin receptor substrate 1 (IRS-1) or by the adapter protein Shc; in insulin-resistant states, phosphorylation of IRS-1 on tyrosine residue is impaired, while Shc activation remains intact [6].

5. Insulin action in skeletal muscle and adipose tissue

Insulin acts as the master regulator of glucose metabolism, with one of its major actions being the increase in glucose uptake by skeletal muscle and adipose tissue. This process involves the translocation of the polypeptide called glucose transporter type 4 (GLUT4) into the plasma membrane of myocytes and adipocytes. Within minutes of insulin binding to its receptor, cytoplasmic vesicles containing GLUT4 (constituting a specialized intracellular organelle called "GLUT4 storage vesicles" or GSVs) translocate from the cytoplasm to the cell surface, fuse their membrane with the plasma membrane, and insert GLUT4 glucose transporters into the plasma membrane, thus permitting glucose uptake [80]. GLUT4 translocation is finely regulated at several stages, and this process does not involve the internalization of the insulin-IR complex.

The GLUT4 storage compartment is in dynamic communication with general recycling endosomes, thus generating a steady-state whereby ~90–95% of GLUT4 resides intracellularly at any point in time in both adipose and muscle cells [2, 81]. In muscle and adipose cells, insulin binds to IR on the cell surface, promotes the IR tyrosine kinase activity toward autophosphorylation, and activates the downstream insulin signaling cascade to PI3K and Akt, which results in the dynamic remodeling of cortical actin filaments and rapid mobilization of GSVs from perinuclear/cytosolic depots toward the cell periphery; this mobilization ultimately allows GSV tethering, docking, and fusion with the plasma membrane [2, 82]. Reduced GLUT4 translocation to the plasma membrane has been described in skeletal muscle of diabetic rodents and humans as a consequence of defects in the insulin-mediated signals promoting GLUT4 vesicle release from the GSV organelle and GLUT4 vesicle interaction-fusion with the plasma membrane [83, 84].

The GLUT4 transporter is expressed in all insulin-sensitive tissues, including adipose tissue and skeletal and cardiac muscle [6, 85]. On the other hand, GLUT1 is insulin-insensitive and represents the basal glucose transporter in adipose tissue, skeletal muscle, erythrocytes, and the brain. Glucose transporter type 2 (GLUT2) is the major glucose transporter required for glucose sensing and hepatic glucose uptake and output; it is the major member of the GLUT family in pancreatic beta cells and hepatocytes, but it is also abundant in the intestine and kidney [6, 86].

Approximately 60–70% of the ingested glucose load escapes the hepatic glucose uptake and is disposed of (under the insulin action) by muscle and other obligate glucose utilizers such as smooth muscle, CNS, and formed blood elements, with about two-thirds of the glucose entering the glycogen synthetic pathway and about one-third entering the glycolytic pathway [6, 87]. Quantitatively, the glucose uptake by adipose tissue accounts for about 5–10% of the ingested glucose load [6].

5.1 Insulin action in skeletal muscle

Skeletal muscle represents the body's largest reservoir of carbohydrate and protein. Therefore, it is highly dependent on the insulin-mediated uptake of glucose and amino acids to sustain such intracellular nutrient pools [6]. Following a meal, approximately 60–70% of the ingested carbohydrate is disposed of (under the insulin action) by skeletal muscle, highlighting the critical role of insulin-mediated muscle glucose uptake in postprandial glycemic control [6, 88].

In skeletal muscle, insulin binds to the extracellular domain (α subunits) of the IR expressed on the myocellular membrane. This binding leads to the transphosphorylation of the intracellular IR β subunits and to the tyrosine phosphorylation of IRS proteins [6, 89, 90]. Then, phosphorylated IRS-1 activates PI3K, leading to the generation of phosphatidylinositol 3,4,5-trisphosphate (PIP3) and subsequent phosphorylation and activation of Akt, that ultimately stimulates GLUT4 translocation from the intracellular GSV organelle to the plasma membrane [6, 91].

In myocytes, insulin upregulates the transcription and activity of the enzyme hexokinase II. This enzyme catalyzes the intracellular phosphorylation of glucose to G6P [92–94], which is readily utilized for the synthesis and storage of glycogen and conversion into pyruvate via the glycolytic pathway. Insulin activates the enzyme pyruvate dehydrogenase, which transforms pyruvate into acetyl-CoA. Skeletal muscle glycolysis is primarily driven by the rate of acetyl-CoA generation in the mitochondria [6, 95]. The increase in intracellular concentration of G6P also promotes glycogen synthesis (especially in the presence of sustained muscle glucose uptake), since G6P acts as a major allosteric activator of glycogen synthesis via inhibition of glycogen phosphorylase and activation of glycogen synthase [96, 97]. Impairment in insulin-induced hexokinase II expression has been suggested to contribute to insulin resistance in obesity and T2DM [98].

According to its anabolic actions, insulin plays an essential role in the regulation of muscle protein metabolism and maintenance of skeletal muscle mass by suppressing muscle proteolysis (through the inactivation of autophagy mediated by Akt) and by stimulating muscle protein synthesis (via activation of the mammalian target of rapamycin complex 1, a key effector of cellular protein synthesis) [6, 99]. After ingesting a meal, the increase in circulating amino acid concentrations allows for the net stimulation of muscle protein synthesis induced by the postprandial rise in circulating insulin levels [6, 100].

5.2 Insulin action in adipose tissue

Adipose tissue represents the major storage site of fatty acids, which are released in the circulation in the form of FFAs after the process called "lipolysis", which consists of the hydrolysis of triglycerides within the adipocytes. During fasting conditions, lipolysis allows for the use of FFAs as an energy source for peripheral tissues. Insulin plays a crucial role in adipose tissue metabolism by stimulating glucose uptake, inhibiting lipolysis (in a dose-response manner), and promoting lipogenesis (with subsequent storage of triglycerides in adipocytes) [6]. FFAs are transported into adipocytes by the scavenger receptor CD36, while glucose is transported into adipocytes by GLUT1 (insulin-independent) and GLUT-4 (insulin-dependent) transporters. The intracellular glucose is then used to synthesize glycerol-3-phosphate (G3P), which is necessary for triglyceride synthesis. Indeed, triglyceride synthesis starts with the generation of diacylglycerols (DAG) from the conversion of glucose into G3P and the binding of two fatty acid acyl-CoA molecules [6].

It has been shown that GLUT4 expression is reduced in insulin-resistant patients with obesity and T2DM [101], thus explaining the reduced glucose uptake observed in visceral and subcutaneous fat of insulin-resistant subjects [6].

In adipocytes, insulin binds to IR leading to tyrosine phosphorylation and activation of the IR, resulting in the interaction with IRS-1 and IRS-2 and subsequent activation of the PI3K complex [6]. Insulin-mediated activation of PKB promotes the activation of the mammalian target of rapamycin complex 1 (mTORC1), which ultimately results in the inhibition of the adipose triglyceride lipase (ATGL). The enzyme ATGL stimulates the hydrolysis of triglycerides to DAG, with subsequent release of one fatty acid molecule. Insulin also inhibits, via a PKB/Akt-dependent action, the subsequent steps of lipolysis by reducing the activity of the enzyme hormone-sensitive lipase (HSL), which hydrolyzes DAG to monoacylglycerol (MAG) with the release of one fatty acid molecule [6, 102].

In patients with obesity and/or insulin resistance, a resistance to the antilipolytic effect of insulin leads to a chronic increase in circulating levels of FFAs under fasting and fed conditions (despite the postprandial hyperinsulinemia). The chronic increase in circulating FFA levels causes detrimental effects via lipid accumulation in non-adipose tissues such as liver, skeletal muscle, heart, kidney and pancreatic beta cells (a phenomenon known as "lipotoxicity"), and potentially leads to the development of T2DM [103–105].

6. Insulin action in the brain

The brain relies on glucose as its major fuel. Glucose is transported across the cell membranes by facilitated diffusion mediated by two main glucose transporter proteins (GLUT1 and GLUT3) that are differentially expressed in brain endothelial cells, astrocytes, and neurons [106]. The glucose transport into most neurons depends on glucose transporter type 3 (GLUT3). In contrast, the glia and brain endothelial cells depend on GLUT1 activity for glucose uptake from brain interstitial fluid and plasma, respectively [107]. As insulin is not needed for GLUT1- or GLUT3-mediated glucose transport, it is not required for glucose transport into most brain cells [108]. Therefore, the brain and the CNS have long been considered "insulin insensitive and unresponsive." However, evidence from the last two decades has supported that the brain is an insulin-responsive organ and that insulin exerts neuroregulatory properties and additional pleiotropic actions in the CNS [109]. First, insulin can cross the blood-brain barrier via a receptor-mediated process [110], thus achieving concentrations in the cerebrospinal fluid that are approximately one-third of those in the systemic circulation. In the CNS, insulin primarily regulates appetite and energy expenditure by decreasing the expression of the two orexigenic neuropeptides, namely neuropeptide Y (NPY) and agouti-related peptide (AGRP)—released by the same set of neurons within the arcuate nucleus of the hypothalamus—and by increasing the expression of the anorexigenic polypeptide pro-opiomelanocortin (POMC) [111–113].

Growing evidence over the past decade has also shed light on insulin's function in the brain as an important regulator of mood, memory, and cognition, in light of the trophic and developmental actions of insulin on neurons and glial cells. In this regard, accumulating evidence suggests that intranasal insulin administration may represent a valid therapeutic option to improve cognitive function in neurodegenerative diseases by means of its ability to increase cerebral insulin levels and reverse brain insulin resistance [114–117]. Indeed, defects in brain insulin action and altered insulin receptor signaling have emerged as potential contributors to Alzheimer's disease pathophysiology, so this condition has also been termed "type 3 diabetes" [118, 119]. Defects in insulin signaling also provide a link between diabetes and CNS disorders through direct neuronal effects and regulation of mitochondrial function, cholesterol synthesis, tau phosphorylation, and amyloid-beta peptide (Aβ) processing [117, 120].

In the brain, insulin also influences body temperature control, since insulin or IGF-1 injection into the preoptic area of the hypothalamus can activate brown adipose tissue and induce hyperthermia. This effect is lost in neuron-specific IR knockout (NIRKO) mice, suggesting that it is mediated by IR [121]. Studies in NIRKO mice have also shown that insulin acts in the brain to regulate the counterregulatory response to hypoglycemia by directly altering glucose sensing in hypothalamic neurons and shifting the glycemic levels necessary to evoke a normal sympathoadrenal response [122]. Yet, the exact cellular mechanisms underlying all the abovementioned actions of insulin in the CNS remain to be elucidated.

7. Brief overview of systemic insulin actions following postprandial insulin secretion

Insulin is the paramount anabolic hormone promoting carbon energy storage in adipose tissue, skeletal muscle, and liver. As such, insulin represents the master regulator of glucose, lipid, and protein metabolism. Following glucose ingestion, there is a rise in plasma glucose concentrations and subsequent glucose-mediated stimulation of insulin secretion by pancreatic beta cells. The resultant hyperglycemia and hyperinsulinemia determine a series of closely coordinated metabolic responses that return the plasma glucose concentration to normal values within 2 hours, namely: a) inhibition of glucagon secretion from pancreatic alpha cells and direct suppression of endogenous glucose production (mainly HGP); b) inhibition of lipolysis and subsequent decline in plasma FFA and glycerol concentrations, which results in the indirect suppression of HGP and augmented muscle glucose uptake (as FFAs promote HGP and inhibit muscle glucose uptake) [123]; c) stimulation of glucose uptake by myocytes, hepatocytes, and adipocytes; d) skeletal muscle vasodilation contributing to enhanced muscle glucose disposal [6].

8. The role of the kidney in insulin degradation and excretion

Kidneys represent the final "station" of the insulin journey, since they are involved in the last steps of degradation and excretion of the remaining circulating insulin that has not previously been degraded by the liver and that has exerted its peripheral actions. Insulin has a short plasma half-life (about 4–6 minutes), as it is expected from the need to respond rapidly to changes in blood glucose levels [124, 125]. Insulin uptake and degradation represent features of all insulin-sensitive tissues, where the hormone is slowly internalized by cells (such as adipocytes and myocytes) and is then transported to lysosomes for degradation [2]. As it has previously been mentioned, the liver is the primary site of insulin clearance, where approximately 50% of insulin is degraded in the first-pass hepatic clearance and 25% of insulin is degraded in the second-pass hepatic clearance. The clearance of the remaining 25% of undegraded insulin initially released from the pancreas occurs in the kidneys.

Insulin clearance by the kidney occurs via two main mechanisms: i) glomerular filtration and ii) proximal tubular reabsorption and degradation [50, 126]. Glomerular clearance of insulin occurs through both nonspecific diffusion and specific receptor-mediated transport. Thus, insulin is freely filtered across the capillaries of the glomerulus (given its molecular weight of 5808 Da), enters the luminal space, and reaches the proximal tubule. Then, more than 99% of the filtered insulin is reabsorbed by proximal tabular epithelial cells mainly *via* endocytosis (possibly mediated by scavenger receptors such as megalin) [127]. In contrast, less than 1% of filtered insulin appears in the final urine [2, 50]. After being internalized into the proximal tabular epithelial cells, insulin dissociates from its binding sites and proceeds to lysosomes for degradation. Renal insulin clearance also occurs through tubular secretory clearance from post-glomerular, peritubular capillaries via receptor-mediated processes. In particular, IRs expressed on the contraluminal membrane of the epithelial cells (particularly those lining the distal convoluted tubule of the nephron) bind insulin (that comes via diffusion from peritubular capillaries) and transport the hormone intracellularly for degradation [128, 129].

Renal clearance of insulin amounts to approximately 200 mL/min, significantly exceeding the normal glomerular filtration rate (GFR) of 120 mL/min because of the contribution of tubular secretion [130]. It has been proposed that 6 to 8 units of insulin are degraded by the kidneys each day via the two abovementioned mechanisms; this amount accounts for about 25% of the daily pancreatic insulin production [130]. In diabetic patients treated with insulin therapy, the contribution of renal insulin metabolism is even higher than that of non-diabetic subjects or non-insulin-treated diabetic patients, as exogenous insulin enters the systemic circulation directly, without undergoing the first-pass metabolism in the liver. On the other hand, advanced chronic kidney disease (as can be observed in diabetic nephropathy) unavoidably alters the renal insulin clearance and prolongs the half-life of circulating insulin (although a certain degree of insulin resistance may also be present in the early stages of chronic kidney disease) [131]. This often leads to a substantial reduction in the daily insulin requirements of diabetic patients treated with exogenous insulin [131], thus highlighting the importance of renal insulin clearance as a mechanism to regulate insulin's plasma half-life and end the insulin action.

Besides playing a pivotal role in the clearance and degradation of circulating insulin, the kidneys also represent an important site of insulin action. Indeed, IRs expressed on the renal tubular epithelial cells act as sites sensing insulin and promoting important insulin functions, such as inhibition of renal gluconeogenesis, upregulation of renal sodium-glucose co-transporter 2 (SGLT2) protein expression, and reabsorption of sodium, phosphate, and glucose [129, 132]. As it has previously been mentioned, kidneys also contribute to gluconeogenesis, although to a lesser extent compared to the liver. It is now established that, under postabsorptive conditions, 80–90% of the basal rate of endogenous glucose production comes from the liver, with the remaining 10–20% coming from the kidneys [6, 133]. Accordingly, potential factors that explain the increased risk of hypoglycemia observed in chronic kidney disease include reduced renal insulin clearance, decreased caloric intake, impaired release of the counterregulatory hormone epinephrine (due to autonomic neuropathy), concurrent liver failure, reduced metabolism of substances and drugs that can cause a reduction in plasma glucose levels (e.g., alcohol, nonselective beta-blockers, disopyramide), and reduced renal gluconeogenesis [131, 134]. Similar to its action in the liver, insulin suppresses renal gluconeogenesis [135]. However, insulin-resistant states (like T2DM) can cause an impairment of insulin actions in the kidney, leading to increased renal gluconeogenesis [133]. **Figure 2** illustrates the insulin journey in the human body across the "insulin highway."

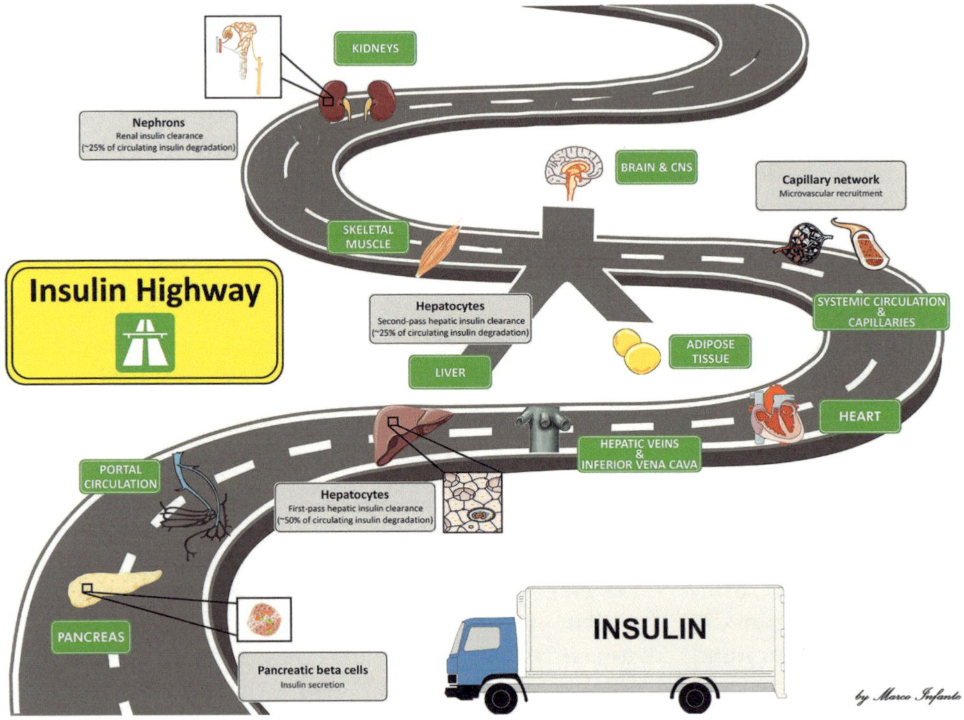

Figure 2.
The insulin journey in the human body across the "insulin highway." Abbreviations: CNS, central nervous system. The figure was conceived by Marco Infante and was partly created with images adapted from Servier Medical Art licensed under a creative commons attribution 3.0 Unported license (https://smart.servier.com/). Digital figure drawing by Enzo Luchetti.

9. Conclusions

Insulin is the paramount anabolic hormone acting as the master regulator of glucose, lipid, and protein metabolism. During fasting and fed states, insulin regulates the flux of nutrients such as glucose, FFAs and amino acids, between liver, skeletal muscle and adipose tissue to ensure a proper nutrient supply to cells and maintain normal glucose homeostasis. Understanding the sequential stages of the physiologic journey of insulin in the human body is pivotal to comprehending the clinical consequences of derangements of insulin secretion and action. Indeed, defects in one or more of such stages can be associated with the development of insulin resistance, metabolic syndrome, and T2DM. Moreover, a thorough knowledge of the insulin bodily journey can assist clinicians in therapeutic decision-making for diabetic patients on exogenous insulin therapy in different clinical settings. The abovementioned stages include the following: i) insulin synthesis and release from pancreatic beta cells; ii) insulin first-pass metabolism and partial clearance in the liver; iii) insulin action on the vasculature and exit from the capillary beds; iv) insulin action in peripheral and central target tissues (skeletal muscle, adipose tissue, liver, and CNS); v) final insulin degradation in the kidney. Each of these stages is finely regulated by complex intracellular mechanisms that take place in different tissues and allow for the anabolic actions of insulin. Yet, several cellular and molecular aspects of the insulin bodily journey are still not entirely clear and need to be elucidated.

Acknowledgements

I would like to thank Mr. Enzo Luchetti for his thorough work in creating the digital figure drawing (**Figure 2**).

Conflict of interest

The author declares no conflict of interest.

Author details

Marco Infante[1,2,3,4*]

1 Department of Systems Medicine, University of Rome Tor Vergata, Rome, Italy

2 Cell Transplant Center, Diabetes Research Institute (DRI), University of Miami Miller School of Medicine, Miami, FL, USA

3 Section of Diabetes and Metabolic Disorders, UniCamillus, Saint Camillus International University of Health Sciences, Rome, Italy

4 Network of Immunity in Infection, Malignancy and Autoimmunity (NIIMA), Universal Scientific Education and Research Network (USERN), Rome, Italy

*Address all correspondence to: marco.infante@uniroma2.it; marco.infante@unicamillus.org and mxi239@miami.edu

References

[1] Gerstein HC, Rutty CJ. Insulin therapy: The discovery that shaped a century. Canadian Journal of Diabetes. 2021;**45**(8):798-803

[2] Tokarz VL, MacDonald PE, Klip A. The cell biology of systemic insulin function. The Journal of Cell Biology. 2018;**217**(7):2273-2289

[3] Taniguchi CM, Emanuelli B, Kahn CR. Critical nodes in signalling pathways: Insights into insulin action. Nature Reviews. Molecular Cell Biology. 2006;7(2):85-96

[4] Odegaard JI, Chawla A. Pleiotropic actions of insulin resistance and inflammation in metabolic homeostasis. Science. 2013;**339**(6116):172-177

[5] Haider N, Lebastchi J, Jayavelu AK, Batista TM, Pan H, Dreyfuss JM, et al. Signaling defects associated with insulin resistance in nondiabetic and diabetic individuals and modification by sex. The Journal of Clinical Investigation. 2021;**131**(21):e151818

[6] Norton L, Shannon C, Gastaldelli A, DeFronzo RA. Insulin: The master regulator of glucose metabolism. Metabolism. 2022;**129**:155142

[7] Isomaa B, Almgren P, Tuomi T, Forsén B, Lahti K, Nissén M, et al. Cardiovascular morbidity and mortality associated with the metabolic syndrome. Diabetes Care. 2001;**24**(4):683-689

[8] Andrali SS, Sampley ML, Vanderford NL, Ozcan S. Glucose regulation of insulin gene expression in pancreatic beta-cells. The Biochemical Journal. 2008;**415**(1):1-10

[9] Lee J, Pilch PF. The insulin receptor: Structure, function, and signaling. The American Journal of Physiology. 1994;**266**(2 Pt 1):C319-C334

[10] Seino S, Seino M, Bell GI. Human insulin-receptor gene. Diabetes. 1990;**39**(2):129-133

[11] Shaw LM. The insulin receptor substrate (IRS) proteins: at the intersection of metabolism and cancer. Cell Cycle. 2011;**10**(11):1750-1756

[12] Goodge KA, Hutton JC. Translational regulation of proinsulin biosynthesis and proinsulin conversion in the pancreatic beta-cell. Seminars in Cell & Developmental Biology. 2000;**11**(4):235-242

[13] Lemaire K, Ravier MA, Schraenen A, Creemers JW, Van de Plas R, Granvik M, et al. Insulin crystallization depends on zinc transporter ZnT8 expression, but is not required for normal glucose homeostasis in mice. Proceedings of the National Academy of Sciences of the United States of America. 2009;**106**(35):14872-14877

[14] Gaisano HY. Recent new insights into the role of SNARE and associated proteins in insulin granule exocytosis. Diabetes, Obesity & Metabolism. 2017;**19**(Suppl 1):115-123

[15] Liang T, Qin T, Xie L, Dolai S, Zhu D, Prentice KJ, et al. New roles of Syntaxin-1A in insulin granule exocytosis and replenishment. The Journal of Biological Chemistry. 2017;**292**(6):2203-2216

[16] Mezza T, Ferraro PM, Sun VA, Moffa S, Cefalo CMA, Quero G, et al. Increased β-cell workload modulates proinsulin-to-insulin ratio in humans. Diabetes. 2018;**67**(11):2389-2396

[17] Sims EK, Chaudhry Z, Watkins R, Syed F, Blum J, Ouyang F, et al. Elevations in the fasting serum proinsulin-to-C-peptide ratio precede the onset of type 1 diabetes. Diabetes Care. 2016;**39**(9):1519-1526

[18] Then C, Gar C, Thorand B, Huth C, Then H, Meisinger C, et al. Proinsulin to insulin ratio is associated with incident type 2 diabetes but not with vascular complications in the KORA F4/FF4 study. BMJ Open Diabetes Research & Care. 2020;**8**(1):e001425

[19] Infante M, Alejandro R, Fabbri A, Ricordi C. The heterogeneity of type 1 diabetes: From immunopathology to immune intervention. In: Chapter 5 in: Translational Autoimmunity (Elsevier). 1st ed. Vol. 4. Autoimmune Diseases in Different Organs. Amsterdam, Netherlands: Elsevier; 2022. DOI: 10.1016/B978-0-12-824466-1.00001-7 ISBN: 9780128244661

[20] Leighton E, Sainsbury CA, Jones GC. A practical review of C-peptide testing in diabetes. Diabetes Therapy. 2017;**8**(3):475-487

[21] Rorsman P, Eliasson L, Renström E, Gromada J, Barg S, Göpel S. The cell physiology of biphasic insulin secretion. News in Physiological Sciences. 2000;**15**:72-77

[22] Parsons TD, Coorssen JR, Horstmann H, Almers W. Docked granules, the exocytic burst, and the need for ATP hydrolysis in endocrine cells. Neuron. 1995;**15**(5):1085-1096

[23] Gerich JE. Is reduced first-phase insulin release the earliest detectable abnormality in individuals destined to develop type 2 diabetes? Diabetes. 2002;**51**(Suppl. 1):S117-S121

[24] Wang Z, Thurmond DC. Mechanisms of biphasic insulin-granule exocytosis - roles of the cytoskeleton, small GTPases and SNARE proteins. Journal of Cell Science. 2009;**122**(Pt 7): 893-903

[25] McCulloch LJ, van de Bunt M, Braun M, Frayn KN, Clark A, Gloyn AL. GLUT2 (SLC2A2) is not the principal glucose transporter in human pancreatic beta cells: Implications for understanding genetic association signals at this locus. Molecular Genetics and Metabolism. 2011;**104**(4):648-653

[26] Rorsman P, Braun M, Zhang Q. Regulation of calcium in pancreatic α- and β-cells in health and disease. Cell Calcium. 2012;**51**(3-4):300-308

[27] Fu Z, Gilbert ER, Liu D. Regulation of insulin synthesis and secretion and pancreatic Beta-cell dysfunction in diabetes. Current Diabetes Reviews. 2013;**9**(1):25-53

[28] Zarkovic M, Henquin JC. Synchronization and entrainment of cytoplasmic Ca2+ oscillations in cell clusters prepared from single or multiple mouse pancreatic islets. American Journal of Physiology. Endocrinology and Metabolism. 2004;**287**(2):E340-E347

[29] Ravier MA, Güldenagel M, Charollais A, Gjinovci A, Caille D, Söhl G, et al. Loss of connexin36 channels alters beta-cell coupling, islet synchronization of glucose-induced Ca2+ and insulin oscillations, and basal insulin release. Diabetes. 2005;**54**(6):1798-1807

[30] Gylfe E, Grapengiesser E, Dansk H, Hellman B. The neurotransmitter ATP triggers Ca2+ responses promoting coordination of pancreatic islet oscillations. Pancreas. 2012;**41**(2): 258-263

[31] Satin LS, Butler PC, Ha J, Sherman AS. Pulsatile insulin secretion,

impaired glucose tolerance and type 2 diabetes. Molecular Aspects of Medicine. 2015;**42**:61-77

[32] Tang SC, Baeyens L, Shen CN, Peng SJ, Chien HJ, Scheel DW, et al. Human pancreatic neuro-insular network in health and fatty infiltration. Diabetologia. 2018;**61**(1):168-181

[33] Del Prato S, Leonetti F, Simonson DC, Sheehan P, Matsuda M, DeFronzo RA. Effect of sustained physiologic hyperinsulinaemia and hyperglycaemia on insulin secretion and insulin sensitivity in man. Diabetologia. 1994;**37**(10):1025-1035

[34] Song SH, McIntyre SS, Shah H, Veldhuis JD, Hayes PC, Butler PC. Direct measurement of pulsatile insulin secretion from the portal vein in human subjects. The Journal of Clinical Endocrinology and Metabolism. 2000;**85**(12):4491-4499

[35] Pørksen N, Munn S, Steers J, Vore S, Veldhuis J, Butler P. Pulsatile insulin secretion accounts for 70% of total insulin secretion during fasting. The American Journal of Physiology. 1995;**269**(3 Pt 1):E478-E488

[36] Matveyenko AV, Liuwantara D, Gurlo T, Kirakossian D, Dalla Man C, Cobelli C, et al. Pulsatile portal vein insulin delivery enhances hepatic insulin action and signaling. Diabetes. 2012;**61**(9):2269-2279

[37] Meier JJ, Veldhuis JD, Butler PC. Pulsatile insulin secretion dictates systemic insulin delivery by regulating hepatic insulin extraction in humans. Diabetes. 2005;**54**(6):1649-1656

[38] Horwitz DL, Starr JI, Mako ME, Blackard WG, Rubenstein AH. Proinsulin, insulin, and C-peptide concentrations in human portal and peripheral blood. The Journal of Clinical Investigation. 1975;**55**(6):1278-1283

[39] Braet F, Wisse E. Structural and functional aspects of liver sinusoidal endothelial cell fenestrae: A review. Comparative Hepatology. 2002;**1**(1):1

[40] Najjar SM, Perdomo G. Hepatic insulin clearance: Mechanism and physiology. Physiology (Bethesda, Md.). 2019;**34**(3):198-215

[41] Carpentier JL, Fehlmann M, Van Obberghen E, Gorden P, Orci L. Redistribution of 125I-insulin on the surface of rat hepatocytes as a function of dissociation time. Diabetes. 1985;**34**(10):1002-1007

[42] Hall C, Yu H, Choi E. Insulin receptor endocytosis in the pathophysiology of insulin resistance. Experimental & Molecular Medicine. 2020;**52**(6):911-920

[43] Fehlmann M, Carpentier JL, Le Cam A, Thamm P, Saunders D, Brandenburg D, et al. Biochemical and morphological evidence that the insulin receptor is internalized with insulin in hepatocytes. The Journal of Cell Biology. 1982;**93**(1):82-87

[44] Goodner CJ, Sweet IR, Harrison HC. Rapid reduction and return of surface insulin receptors after exposure to brief pulses of insulin in perifused rat hepatocytes. Diabetes. 1988;**37**(10):1316-1323

[45] Michael MD, Kulkarni RN, Postic C, Previs SF, Shulman GI, Magnuson MA, et al. Loss of insulin signaling in hepatocytes leads to severe insulin resistance and progressive hepatic dysfunction. Molecular Cell. 2000;**6**(1):87-97

[46] Horst AK, Najjar SM, Wagener C, Tiegs G. CEACAM1 in liver injury,

metabolic and immune regulation. International Journal of Molecular Sciences. 2018;**19**(10):3110

[47] Poy MN, Yang Y, Rezaei K, Fernström MA, Lee AD, Kido Y, et al. CEACAM1 regulates insulin clearance in liver. Nature Genetics. 2002;**30**(3):270-276

[48] Yokono K, Roth RA, Baba S. Identification of insulin-degrading enzyme on the surface of cultured human lymphocytes, rat hepatoma cells, and primary cultures of rat hepatocytes. Endocrinology. 1982;**111**(4):1102-1108

[49] Eaton RP, Allen RC, Schade DS. Hepatic removal of insulin in normal man: Dose response to endogenous insulin secretion. The Journal of Clinical Endocrinology and Metabolism. 1983;**56**(6):1294-1300

[50] Duckworth WC, Bennett RG, Hamel FG. Insulin degradation: progress and potential. Endocrine Reviews. 1998;**19**(5):608-624

[51] Jung SH, Jung CH, Reaven GM, Kim SH. Adapting to insulin resistance in obesity: Role of insulin secretion and clearance. Diabetologia. 2018;**61**(3):681-687

[52] Lee W. The CEACAM1 expression is decreased in the liver of severely obese patients with or without diabetes. Diagnostic Pathology. 2011;**6**:40

[53] Santoleri D, Titchenell PM. Resolving the paradox of hepatic insulin resistance. Cellular and Molecular Gastroenterology and Hepatology. 2019;7(2):447-456

[54] Hatting M, Tavares CDJ, Sharabi K, Rines AK, Puigserver P. Insulin regulation of gluconeogenesis. Annals of the New York Academy of Sciences. 2018;**1411**(1):21-35

[55] Jiang G, Zhang BB. Glucagon and regulation of glucose metabolism. American Journal of Physiology. Endocrinology and Metabolism. 2003;**284**(4):E671-E678

[56] Rui L. Energy metabolism in the liver. Comprehensive Physiology. 2014;**4**(1):177-197

[57] Kaneko K, Shirotani T, Araki E, Matsumoto K, Taguchi T, Motoshima H, et al. Insulin inhibits glucagon secretion by the activation of PI3-kinase in In-R1-G9 cells. Diabetes Research and Clinical Practice. 1999;**44**(2):83-92

[58] Perry RJ, Zhang D, Guerra MT, Brill AL, Goedeke L, Nasiri AR, et al. Glucagon stimulates gluconeogenesis by INSP3R1-mediated hepatic lipolysis. Nature. 2020;**579**(7798):279-283

[59] Legouis D, Faivre A, Cippà PE, de Seigneux S. Renal gluconeogenesis: An underestimated role of the kidney in systemic glucose metabolism. Nephrology, Dialysis, Transplantation. 26 Jul 2022;**37**(8):1417-1425

[60] Vily-Petit J, Soty-Roca M, Silva M, Raffin M, Gautier-Stein A, Rajas F, et al. Intestinal gluconeogenesis prevents obesity-linked liver steatosis and non-alcoholic fatty liver disease. Gut. 2020;**69**(12):2193-2202

[61] Argilés JM, Campos N, Lopez-Pedrosa JM, Rueda R, Rodriguez-Mañas L. Skeletal muscle regulates metabolism via Interorgan crosstalk: Roles in health and disease. Journal of the American Medical Directors Association. 2016;**17**(9):789-796

[62] Yip J, Geng X, Shen J, Ding Y. Cerebral gluconeogenesis and diseases. Frontiers in Pharmacology. 2016;7:521

[63] Nakae J, Kitamura T, Silver DL, Accili D. The forkhead transcription

factor Foxo1 (Fkhr) confers insulin sensitivity onto glucose-6-phosphatase expression. The Journal of Clinical Investigation. 2001;**108**(9):1359-1367

[64] Streeper RS, Svitek CA, Chapman S, Greenbaum LE, Taub R, O'Brien RM. A multicomponent insulin response sequence mediates a strong repression of mouse glucose-6-phosphatase gene transcription by insulin. The Journal of Biological Chemistry. 1997;**272**(18):11698-11701

[65] Sasaki K, Cripe TP, Koch SR, Andreone TL, Petersen DD, Beale EG, et al. Multihormonal regulation of phosphoenolpyruvate carboxykinase gene transcription. The dominant role of insulin. The Journal of Biological Chemistry. 1984;**259**(24):15242-15251

[66] Feliú JE, Hue L, Hers HG. Hormonal control of pyruvate kinase activity and of gluconeogenesis in isolated hepatocytes. Proceedings of the National Academy of Sciences of the United States of America. 1976;**73**(8):2762-2766

[67] Sparks JD, Sparks CE. Insulin modulation of hepatic synthesis and secretion of apolipoprotein B by rat hepatocytes. The Journal of Biological Chemistry. 1990;**265**(15):8854-8862

[68] Sparks JD, Sparks CE, Adeli K. Selective hepatic insulin resistance, VLDL overproduction, and hypertriglyceridemia. Arteriosclerosis, Thrombosis, and Vascular Biology. 2012;**32**(9):2104-2112

[69] Zeng G, Nystrom FH, Ravichandran LV, Cong LN, Kirby M, Mostowski H, et al. Roles for insulin receptor, PI3-kinase, and Akt in insulin-signaling pathways related to production of nitric oxide in human vascular endothelial cells. Circulation. 2000;**101**(13):1539-1545

[70] Lee MR, Li L, Kitazawa T. Cyclic GMP causes Ca2+ desensitization in vascular smooth muscle by activating the myosin light chain phosphatase. The Journal of Biological Chemistry. 1997;**272**(8):5063-5068

[71] Barrett EJ, Eggleston EM, Inyard AC, Wang H, Li G, Chai W, et al. The vascular actions of insulin control its delivery to muscle and regulate the rate-limiting step in skeletal muscle insulin action. Diabetologia. 2009;**52**(5):752-764

[72] Vincent MA, Clerk LH, Lindner JR, Klibanov AL, Clark MG, Rattigan S, et al. Microvascular recruitment is an early insulin effect that regulates skeletal muscle glucose uptake in vivo. Diabetes. 2004;**53**(6):1418-1423

[73] Bonadonna RC, Saccomani MP, Seely L, Zych KS, Ferrannini E, Cobelli C, et al. Glucose transport in human skeletal muscle. The in vivo response to insulin. Diabetes. 1993;**42**(1):191-198

[74] Keske MA, Clerk LH, Price WJ, Jahn LA, Barrett EJ. Obesity blunts microvascular recruitment in human forearm muscle after a mixed meal. Diabetes Care. 2009;**32**(9):1672-1677

[75] de Jongh RT, Serné EH, RG IJ, de Vries G, Stehouwer CD. Impaired microvascular function in obesity: Implications for obesity-associated microangiopathy, hypertension, and insulin resistance. Circulation. 2004;**109**(21):2529-2535

[76] Clerk LH, Vincent MA, Jahn LA, Liu Z, Lindner JR, Barrett EJ. Obesity blunts insulin-mediated microvascular recruitment in human forearm muscle. Diabetes. 2006;**55**(5):1436-1442

[77] Lee WL, Klip A. Endothelial transcytosis of insulin: Does it contribute

to insulin resistance? Physiology (Bethesda, Md.). 2016;**31**(5):336-345

[78] Kashyap SR, Roman LJ, Lamont J, Masters BS, Bajaj M, Suraamornkul S, et al. Insulin resistance is associated with impaired nitric oxide synthase activity in skeletal muscle of type 2 diabetic subjects. The Journal of Clinical Endocrinology and Metabolism. 2005;**90**(2):1100-1105

[79] DeFronzo RA. Insulin resistance, lipotoxicity, type 2 diabetes and atherosclerosis: The missing links. The Claude Bernard lecture 2009. Diabetologia. 2010;**53**(7):1270-1287

[80] Li DT, Habtemichael EN, Julca O, Sales CI, Westergaard XO, DeVries SG, et al. GLUT4 storage vesicles: Specialized organelles for regulated trafficking. The Yale Journal of Biology and Medicine. 2019;**92**(3):453-470

[81] Coster AC, Govers R, James DE. Insulin stimulates the entry of GLUT4 into the endosomal recycling pathway by a quantal mechanism. Traffic. 2004;**5**(10):763-771

[82] Chiu TT, Patel N, Shaw AE, Bamburg JR, Klip A. Arp2/3- and cofilin-coordinated actin dynamics is required for insulin-mediated GLUT4 translocation to the surface of muscle cells. Molecular Biology of the Cell. 2010;**21**(20):3529-3539

[83] Klip A, Ramlal T, Bilan PJ, Cartee GD, Gulve EA, Holloszy JO. Recruitment of GLUT-4 glucose transporters by insulin in diabetic rat skeletal muscle. Biochemical and Biophysical Research Communications. 1990;**172**(2):728-736

[84] Zierath JR, He L, Gumà A, Odegoard Wahlström E, Klip A, Wallberg-Henriksson H. Insulin action on glucose transport and plasma membrane GLUT4 content in skeletal muscle from patients with NIDDM. Diabetologia. 1996;**39**(10):1180-1189

[85] Shao D, Tian R. Glucose transporters in cardiac metabolism and hypertrophy. Comprehensive Physiology. 2015;**6**(1):331-351

[86] Chadt A, Al-Hasani H. Glucose transporters in adipose tissue, liver, and skeletal muscle in metabolic health and disease. Pflügers Archiv. 2020;**472**(9):1273-1298

[87] Thiebaud D, Jacot E, DeFronzo RA, Maeder E, Jequier E, Felber JP. The effect of graded doses of insulin on total glucose uptake, glucose oxidation, and glucose storage in man. Diabetes. 1982;**31**(11):957-963

[88] Kelley D, Mitrakou A, Marsh H, Schwenk F, Benn J, Sonnenberg G, et al. Skeletal muscle glycolysis, oxidation, and storage of an oral glucose load. The Journal of Clinical Investigation. 1988;**81**(5):1563-1571

[89] Jaiswal N, Gavin MG, Quinn WJ, Luongo TS, Gelfer RG, Baur JA, et al. The role of skeletal muscle Akt in the regulation of muscle mass and glucose homeostasis. Molecular Metabolism. 2019;**28**:1-13

[90] Isakoff SJ, Taha C, Rose E, Marcusohn J, Klip A, Skolnik EY. The inability of phosphatidylinositol 3-kinase activation to stimulate GLUT4 translocation indicates additional signaling pathways are required for insulin-stimulated glucose uptake. Proceedings of the National Academy of Sciences of the United States of America. 1995;**92**(22):10247-10251

[91] Ramos PA, Lytle KA, Delivanis D, Nielsen S, LeBrasseur NK, Jensen MD.

Insulin-stimulated muscle glucose uptake and insulin signaling in lean and obese humans. The Journal of Clinical Endocrinology and Metabolism. 2021;**106**(4):e1631-e1e46

[92] Vogt C, Yki-Jarvinen H, Iozzo P, Pipek R, Pendergrass M, Koval J, et al. Effects of insulin on subcellular localization of hexokinase II in human skeletal muscle in vivo. The Journal of Clinical Endocrinology and Metabolism. 1998;**83**(1):230-234

[93] Saccomani MP, Bonadonna RC, Bier DM, DeFronzo RA, Cobelli C. A model to measure insulin effects on glucose transport and phosphorylation in muscle: A three-tracer study. The American Journal of Physiology. 1996;**270**(1 Pt 1):E170-E185

[94] Mandarino LJ, Printz RL, Cusi KA, Kinchington P, O'Doherty RM, Osawa H, et al. Regulation of hexokinase II and glycogen synthase mRNA, protein, and activity in human muscle. The American Journal of Physiology. 1995;**269**(4 Pt 1): E701-E708

[95] Mandarino LJ, Wright KS, Verity LS, Nichols J, Bell JM, Kolterman OG, et al. Effects of insulin infusion on human skeletal muscle pyruvate dehydrogenase, phosphofructokinase, and glycogen synthase. Evidence for their role in oxidative and nonoxidative glucose metabolism. The Journal of Clinical Investigation. 1987;**80**(3):655-663

[96] Villar-Palasí C, Guinovart JJ. The role of glucose 6-phosphate in the control of glycogen synthase. The FASEB Journal. 1997;**11**(7):544-558

[97] Bouskila M, Hunter RW, Ibrahim AF, Delattre L, Peggie M, van Diepen JA, et al. Allosteric regulation of glycogen synthase controls glycogen synthesis in muscle. Cell Metabolism. 2010;**12**(5):456-466

[98] Pendergrass M, Koval J, Vogt C, Yki-Jarvinen H, Iozzo P, Pipek R, et al. Insulin-induced hexokinase II expression is reduced in obesity and NIDDM. Diabetes. 1998;**47**(3):387-394

[99] Gelfand RA, Barrett EJ. Effect of physiologic hyperinsulinemia on skeletal muscle protein synthesis and breakdown in man. The Journal of Clinical Investigation. 1987;**80**(1):1-6

[100] Luzi L, Castellino P, Simonson DC, Petrides AS, DeFronzo RA. Leucine metabolism in IDDM. Role of insulin and substrate availability. Diabetes. 1990;**39**(1):38-48

[101] Garvey WT, Maianu L, Hueckstеadt TP, Birnbaum MJ, Molina JM, Ciaraldi TP. Pretranslational suppression of a glucose transporter protein causes insulin resistance in adipocytes from patients with non-insulin-dependent diabetes mellitus and obesity. The Journal of Clinical Investigation. 1991;**87**(3):1072-1081

[102] Chakrabarti P, Kim JY, Singh M, Shin YK, Kim J, Kumbrink J, et al. Insulin inhibits lipolysis in adipocytes via the evolutionarily conserved mTORC1-Egr1-ATGL-mediated pathway. Molecular and Cellular Biology. 2013;**33**(18):3659-3666

[103] Oh YS, Bae GD, Baek DJ, Park EY, Jun HS. Fatty acid-induced lipotoxicity in pancreatic Beta-cells during development of type 2 diabetes. Frontiers in Endocrinology (Lausanne). 2018;**9**:384

[104] Ye R, Onodera T, Scherer PE. Lipotoxicity and β cell maintenance in obesity and type 2 diabetes. Journal of the Endocrine Society. 2019;**3**(3):617-631

[105] van Herpen NA, Schrauwen-Hinderling VB. Lipid accumulation in non-adipose tissue and lipotoxicity. Physiology & Behavior. 2008;**94**(2):231-241

[106] Duelli R, Kuschinsky W. Brain glucose transporters: Relationship to local energy demand. News in Physiological Sciences. 2001;**16**:71-76

[107] McEwen BS, Reagan LP. Glucose transporter expression in the central nervous system: Relationship to synaptic function. European Journal of Pharmacology. 2004;**490**(1-3):13-24

[108] Gray SM, Meijer RI, Barrett EJ. Insulin regulates brain function, but how does it get there? Diabetes. 2014;**63**(12):3992-3997

[109] Ghasemi R, Haeri A, Dargahi L, Mohamed Z, Ahmadiani A. Insulin in the brain: Sources, localization and functions. Molecular Neurobiology. 2013;**47**(1):145-171

[110] Woods SC, Seeley RJ, Baskin DG, Schwartz MW. Insulin and the blood-brain barrier. Current Pharmaceutical Design. 2003;**9**(10):795-800

[111] Filippi BM, Abraham MA, Yue JT, Lam TK. Insulin and glucagon signaling in the central nervous system. Reviews in Endocrine & Metabolic Disorders. 2013;**14**(4):365-375

[112] Schwartz MW, Woods SC, Porte D, Seeley RJ, Baskin DG. Central nervous system control of food intake. Nature. 2000;**404**(6778):661-671

[113] Schwartz MW, Sipols AJ, Marks JL, Sanacora G, White JD, Scheurink A, et al. Inhibition of hypothalamic neuropeptide Y gene expression by insulin. Endocrinology. 1992;**130**(6):3608-3616

[114] Lee SH, Zabolotny JM, Huang H, Lee H, Kim YB. Insulin in the nervous system and the mind: Functions in metabolism, memory, and mood. Molecular Metabolism. 2016;5(8):589-601

[115] Lv H, Tang L, Guo C, Jiang Y, Gao C, Wang Y, et al. Intranasal insulin administration may be highly effective in improving cognitive function in mice with cognitive dysfunction by reversing brain insulin resistance. Cognitive Neurodynamics. 2020;**14**(3):323-338

[116] Duarte AI, Moreira PI, Oliveira CR. Insulin in central nervous system: More than just a peripheral hormone. Journal of Aging Research. 2012;**2012**:384017

[117] Infante M, Della-Morte D. Diabetes and cognitive dysfunction: A dangerous liaison. CellR4. 2019;7:e2776. DOI: 10.32113/cellr4_201910_2776

[118] Griffith CM, Eid T, Rose GM, Patrylo PR. Evidence for altered insulin receptor signaling in Alzheimer's disease. Neuropharmacology. 2018;**136**(Pt B): 202-215

[119] de la Monte SM, Wands JR. Alzheimer's disease is type 3 diabetes-evidence reviewed. Journal of Diabetes Science and Technology. 2008;**2**(6):1101-1113

[120] Kleinridders A, Ferris HA, Cai W, Kahn CR. Insulin action in brain regulates systemic metabolism and brain function. Diabetes. 2014;**63**(7):2232-2243

[121] Sanchez-Alavez M, Osborn O, Tabarean IV, Holmberg KH, Eberwine J, Kahn CR, et al. Insulin-like growth factor 1-mediated hyperthermia involves anterior hypothalamic insulin receptors. The Journal of Biological Chemistry. 2011;**286**(17):14983-14990

[122] Diggs-Andrews KA, Zhang X, Song Z, Daphna-Iken D, Routh VH, Fisher SJ. Brain insulin action regulates hypothalamic glucose sensing and the counterregulatory response to hypoglycemia. Diabetes. 2010;**59**(9):2271-2280

[123] Bergman RN, Iyer MS. Indirect regulation of endogenous glucose production by insulin: The single gateway hypothesis revisited. Diabetes. 2017;**66**(7):1742-1747

[124] Duckworth WC. Insulin degradation: Mechanisms, products, and significance. Endocrine Reviews. 1988;**9**(3):319-345

[125] Morishima T, Pye S, Bradshaw C, Radziuk J. Posthepatic rate of appearance of insulin: Measurement and validation in the nonsteady state. The American Journal of Physiology. 1992;**263**(4 Pt 1): E772-E779

[126] Hysing J, Tolleshaug H, Kindberg GM. Renal uptake and degradation of trapped-label insulin. Renal Physiology and Biochemistry. 1989;**12**(4):228-237

[127] Christensen EI, Birn H, Verroust P, Moestrup SK. Membrane receptors for endocytosis in the renal proximal tubule. International Review of Cytology. 1998;**180**:237-284

[128] Nielsen S, Nielsen JT, Christensen EI. Luminal and basolateral uptake of insulin in isolated, perfused, proximal tubules. The American Journal of Physiology. 1987;**253**(5 Pt 2): F857-F867

[129] Rabkin R, Ryan MP, Duckworth WC. The renal metabolism of insulin. Diabetologia. 1984;**27**(3):351-357

[130] Palmer BF. Carbohydrate and Insulin Metabolism in Chronic Kidney Disease https://www.uptodate.com/contents/carbohydrate-and-insulin-metabolism-in-chronic-kidney-disease. [Accessed: July 18, 2022]

[131] Sampanis C. Management of hyperglycemia in patients with diabetes mellitus and chronic renal failure. Hippokratia. 2008;**12**(1):22-27

[132] Pereira-Moreira R, Muscelli E. Effect of insulin on proximal tubules handling of glucose: A systematic review. Journal Diabetes Research. 2020;**2020**:8492467

[133] Sharma R, Tiwari S. Renal gluconeogenesis in insulin resistance: A culprit for hyperglycemia in diabetes. World Journal of Diabetes. 2021;**12**(5):556-568

[134] Pecoits-Filho R, Abensur H, Betônico CC, Machado AD, Parente EB, Queiroz M, et al. Interactions between kidney disease and diabetes: Dangerous liaisons. Diabetology and Metabolic Syndrome. 2016;**8**:50

[135] Cersosimo E, Garlick P, Ferretti J. Regulation of splanchnic and renal substrate supply by insulin in humans. Metabolism. 2000;**49**(5):676-683

Chapter 2

Insulin Receptor Isoforms in Physiology and Metabolic Disease

Noah Moruzzi and Francesca Lazzeri-Barcelo

Abstract

Insulin receptors (IRs) are ubiquitously expressed and essential for all cell types. Their signaling cascades are connected to key pathways involved in cell metabolism, proliferation, and differentiation, amongst others. Thus, dysregulation of IR-mediated signaling can lead to diseases such as metabolic disorders. In mammals, the IR pre-mRNA is alternatively spliced to generate two receptor isoforms, IR-A and IR-B, which differ in 12 amino acids in the α-chain involved in ligand binding. Given the isoforms have different affinities for their ligands insulin, proinsulin, and insulin-like growth factors (IGFs), it is speculated that IR amount and splicing regulation might contribute to a change in IR-mediated effects and/or insulin resistance. The aim of this chapter is to increase awareness of this subject in the research fields of diseases characterized by disturbances in insulin signaling. Here, we will describe the IR isoform distribution and discuss the current knowledge of their expression and ligand binding affinities as well as their signaling in physiology and during obesity and type 2 diabetes in humans and animal models. Moreover, we will discuss the necessary steps to gain a better understanding on the function and regulation of the IR isoforms, which could result in future therapeutic approaches against IR-related dysfunction.

Keywords: insulin receptor isoforms, insulin receptor, IR-A, IR-B, diabetes, obesity, pancreatic islets, insulin signaling, adipose tissue

1. Introduction

In invertebrates, one ancestral gene, DAF-2, encodes one receptor that binds insulin-like peptides [1]. With the emergence of vertebrates, three distinct receptors appeared, namely: the insulin receptor (IR), the type 1 insulin-like growth factor receptor (IGF1R), and an orphan receptor called the insulin receptor-related receptor (IRR). The genes encoding these receptors share similar genomic organization, with conserved α and β protein chains that are synthesized from one single pre-mRNA (reviewed in [2]). While originally all three receptors were formed by 21 exons, both IRR and IR acquired independently one extra exon, namely exon 11. The IRR exon 11 can be traced back to amphibians, whereas IR exon 11 is found exclusively in mammals [3, 4]. Thus, exclusively in mammals, the exon 11 of the IR gene is alternatively spliced to produce two protein isoforms called IR-A and IR-B. To trace the origin of

IR isoforms, Hernández-Sánchez et al. analyzed their transcripts in different species by reverse transcriptase-polymerase chain reaction (RT-PCR) analysis [4]. In mouse tissues, they found tissue-specific expression of both IR-A and IR-B, while in chicken and frog tissues, only the IR-A isoform was detected [4]. The physiological reason for the evolutionary acquisition of the IR-B isoform in mammals is unclear. It seems that the IR-B provided the receptor with higher specificity for insulin and poor binding of other possible ligands of IR-A, which will be discussed later.

2. Characterization of the IR isoforms

2.1 Structure and assembly

In humans, the insulin receptor gene (INSR) maps to human chromosome 19 (in mice, it maps to chromosome 8) and spans more than 120 kb [5]. The insulin receptor complementary DNA (cDNA) was cloned in 1985 by two independent groups [6, 7], giving two different lengths and indicating two isoforms, dependent on the inclusion (IR-B) or exclusion (IR-A) of exon 11. The 36 base pairs of exon 11 (that account for the 12 amino acid difference) encode a portion of the C-terminus of the α-subunit in the vicinity of the ligand-binding domain (reviewed in [8]), resulting in isoform-specific properties of the receptors. A linear α-β amino acid sequence (IR pro-receptor precursor) is translated from the IR mRNA and includes a signal sequence at the N-terminus to enter the endoplasmic reticulum [9]. After cleavage of the signal peptide, the inter-α-chain disulphide dimerization occurs, forming the β-α-α-β structure of the IR [10]. The insulin pro-receptor is further processed in the Golgi apparatus by the protease furin, and the mature IR is then trafficked and inserted in the plasma membrane [11].

The IR and IGF1R belong to the same subgroup of receptor tyrosine kinases and can form either homo-receptors (two IR α-β subunits) or hybrid receptors, consisting of one IR α-β subunit linked to one IGF1R α-β subunit. Furthermore, the two IR splice variants enable the formation of both homo-dimers (IR-A/IR-A) or hetero-dimers (IR-A/IR-B), and similarly, two modalities of hybrid receptor (IR-A/IGF1R and IR-B/IGF1R). Hybrid receptors have been detected in all tissues and cell lines that express both receptor types [12] and it is presumed that both IR-A and IR-B isoforms are equally capable of forming hybrids with IGF1R [13]. The factors regulating their assembly are unknown; however, there is evidence to suggest that the formation of homo-receptors and hybrid receptors is proportional to the relative concentrations of each receptor type [12, 14, 15].

Crystal structures of the IR were determined in 1994 [16] and 2006 [17] and refined in 2016 [18]. Single-particle cryo-electron microscopy has since been used to explore receptor conformations and ligand-receptor complexes [19–21]. It is worth pointing out that these studies used the IR-A isoform to reconstruct and represent the IR. The functional IR consists of two covalently linked IR monomers, that is, two extracellular α-subunits linked by disulphide bonds and two transmembrane-spanning β-subunits. The α-subunit contains either 719 (IR-A) or 731 (IR-B) amino acids and has a molecular mass of approximately 130 kDa. This subunit is entirely extracellular and contains the ligand-binding sites. The transmembrane-spanning β-subunit contains 620 amino acids, has an approximate molecular mass of 95 kDa and is composed by extracellular, transmembrane, and cytosolic domains. The latter domain contains the receptor's tyrosine kinase, which is activated by ligand-binding and conformational change of the IR. Two insulin-binding sites are located in the extracellular α-subunit of the IRs. The primary insulin-binding site (site 1) is formed from elements of the L1 domain and a C-terminal peptide of the α-subunit [22–27]. The second insulin binding site (site 2) has lower ligand binding affinity and is formed from residues in the first and second type III fibronectin repeats [28]. A model for insulin binding to the IR has been showed, in which one single insulin molecule simultaneously engages site 1 of one α-chain and site 2 of the other, thus bridging the two IR monomers; while a second insulin molecule binds to the equivalent, symmetry-related site 1′, creating a second bridging with site 2′. The two insulin molecules effectively crosslink the two IR monomers and thereby activate the IR [8, 20, 21]. As to the possible implications of the differences in the α-chain C-terminal domains of the IR isoforms, comprehending the significance of the 12 extra amino acids is hampered by the lack of structural data using the IR-B isoform. Thus, only secondary structure predictions can be made. It can be inferred that the 12-amino acid fragment of IR-B is most certainly the reason for the lower binding affinity of insulin-like growth factor 1 (IGF1) and insulin-like growth factor 2 (IGF2) toward this receptor isoform in comparison to IR-A (as discussed in Section 2.2). Based on this, Menting et al. speculate that the additional residues in the IR-B α-chain C-terminus are devoid of secondary structure, thus making this structure longer and hindering steric accommodation of these ligands, with a similar situation to be expected regarding insulin binding [29]. Whittaker et al. used alanine-scanning mutagenesis of insulin binding site 1 of IR isoforms A and B transiently expressed in cells to study their insulin binding properties [30]. They found several mutations that compromised insulin binding, some of which produced differential effects between the two receptors, either reducing affinity or inactivating one specific isoform [30].

2.2 Ligand binding affinities of the IR isoforms

The different structures of the IR isoforms are responsible for their functional differences, for example, disparity in ligand affinities, internalization and recycling kinetics, signal transduction, and the activation of specific cellular pathways.

Insulin is the main ligand for the IR, although the receptor also binds IGF1 and IGF2, as well as proinsulin (hormone precursor to insulin) (**Figure 1**). Some groups set out to study the different ligand binding affinities of the IR isoforms and came to different conclusions. To measure isoform-specific ligand binding, the main technique used throughout the different studies was competition for radiolabeled insulin. All studies were conducted using human IR cDNA in mouse or rat cell lines (referred to as hIR-A and hIR-B), probably aiming to translating the findings in humans. Mosthaf et al. expressed hIR-A and hIR-B in Rat-1 cells and found that IR-A had ~2-fold higher affinity for insulin than IR-B, both in intact cells and using detergent solubilized, partially purified receptors [31]. In agreement, Kellerer et al. used partially purified receptors from Rat-1 cells and found that IR-A displayed a higher affinity for insulin compared to IR-B [32]. Accordingly, Yamaguchi et al. also reported a ~2-fold higher affinity for insulin in intact Chinese hamster ovary (CHO) cells expressing hIR-A, in comparison to those expressing hIR-B [33]. A second study by this group found a faster insulin association rate to hIR-A receptors in intact CHO cells, as well as an accelerated insulin dissociation from hIR-B receptors, proposing a biochemical basis for the differential ligand biding affinities [13]. A similar faster dissociation of insulin from hIR-B that could be responsible for the lower affinity of this receptor was shown for Rat-1 cells [34]. To note, contrarily to all studies that used

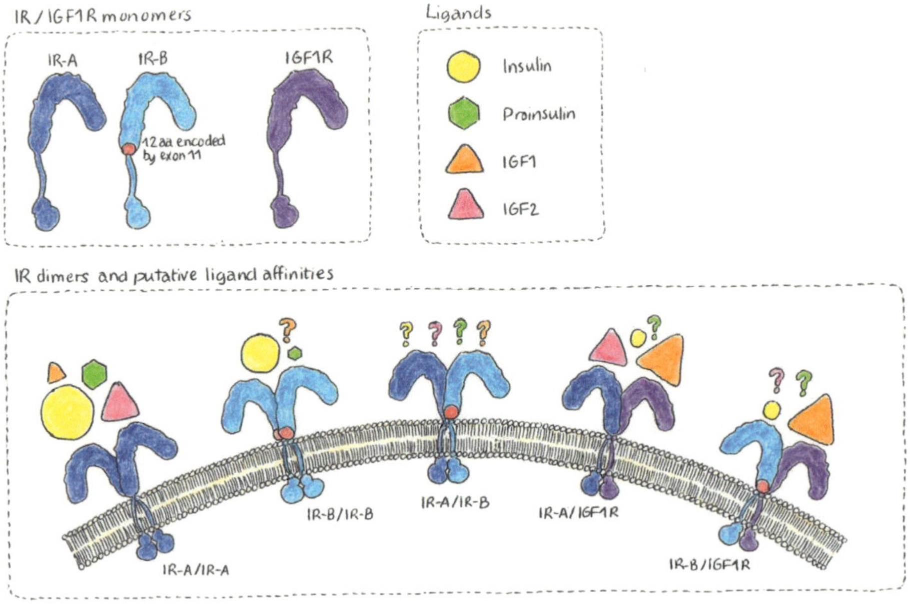

Figure 1.
IR-A, IR-B, and IGF1R monomers, and their combinatorial possibilities of dimerization, with their possible ligands. The size of the different ligands represents the relative affinity for a given receptor. IGF1, insulin-like growth factor 1; IGF1R, type 1 insulin-like growth factor receptor; IGF2, insulin-like growth factor 2; IR, insulin receptor; IR-A, insulin receptor isoform A; IR-B, insulin receptor isoform B.

stimulated native receptors on intact cell membranes, a single work using solubilized recombinant receptors found no significant difference between the affinities of the two IR isoforms for insulin [30].

IR isoform affinities for IGF1 and IGF2 have also been investigated. Frasca et al. used R-cells, a mouse fibroblastic cell line that lack IGF1R, expressing either hIR-A or hIR-B [35]. They reported that IR-A, but not IR-B, binds IGF2 with high affinity (comparable to that of insulin). Further, IGF2 bound to IR-A with similar affinity to that of IGF2 to IGF1R [35]. Using the same cellular system, Sacco et al. reported that IR-A bound IGF2 with high affinity (4-fold lower than that for insulin), whereas IR-A's affinity for IGF1 was 30-fold lower than that for insulin [36]. Proinsulin binding has been less studied compared to the other ligands and its ability to bind differentially the two IR isoforms as well as its possible signal transduction remain an enigma. One study in intact R-cells showed that proinsulin binds and activates both IR isoforms, but had a higher affinity for hIR-A than for hIR-B. Authors report that, similar to IGF2, proinsulin effectively stimulates cell proliferation and migration and curiously had no activity toward IGF1R or IR/IGF1R hybrid receptors [37]. Conversely, McClain's work (mentioned previously) conducted in intact Rat-1 fibroblast cells found that hIR-A and hIR-B bound proinsulin with the same relative affinity [34].

Few studies have addressed the ligand affinities for the different hybrid receptors (IR/IGF1R). Using competition for tracer-labeled insulin and an enzyme-linked immunosorbent assay (ELISA)-based method, Slaaby et al. found that IR-A/IGF1R and IR-B/IGF1R hybrid receptors respond 20 to 50 times more effectively to IGF1 than to insulin [38, 39]. The increase in IGF1R expression and thereby its incorporation into hybrid formation with IR has prompted a potential role of hybrid receptors in reducing cell insulin responsiveness. Studies in CHO cells suggest that hybrids between IGF1R and both IR isoforms have low binding affinity for insulin and high affinity for IGF1 and IGF2 [40]. Another study in R-cells showed that IR-B/IGF1R receptors had high affinity only for IGF1, whereas hybrid IR-A/IGF1R receptors also bound IGF2 and insulin [41].

In summary, the accumulated knowledge suggests that IR-A has higher affinity for insulin, IGF1 and IGF2 compared to IR-B and that hybrid receptors show a preferential affinity for IGF1 (**Figure 1**). This could be due to the availability/inaccessibility of the different binding sites in hybrid receptors. The majority of these affinity studies were conducted using mainly tracer-labeled ligand technique and the works on binding affinity for insulin to IR-A/IR-B are dated more than two decades ago. Molecular chemistry methods have advanced since then and it could be of interest to verify these affinity studies with improved tools comparing primary cells (with double knockout of IR and IGF1R) where only one IR isoform (of the same species of the cells) is expressed at a time. Moreover, ligand binding could potentially be altered by different post-translational modifications of the α-chain such as specific glycosylation patterns and different lipid raft composition, which could both vary between cell types and under different culture conditions.

2.3 Functional differences between the IR isoforms

The IR isoforms seem to display equal receptor activation and kinase activity triggered by the binding of insulin. McClain et al. investigated insulin-stimulated tyrosine kinase activity in solubilized hIR-A and hIR-B receptors by exposure to insulin and radioactive ATP and found similar accumulated radioactivity in the Tyr-phosphorylated receptors [34]. On the contrary, Kellerer et al., preparing equal amounts of solubilized hIR-A and hIR-B, found higher radioactivity for hIR-B (2.5-fold) after stimulation with insulin and phosphorus-32 [32]. However, when performing the same experiment on native receptors in human embryonic kidney (HEK) intact cell membrane transiently expressing the isoforms, they detected no difference in tyrosine kinase activity. Neither did they report differences when they used short-time trypsinization to cleave the α-subunit and activate the tyrosine kinase [32]. The latter data suggests that solubilized receptors were able to undergo different activation compared to receptors integrated in the plasma membrane of intact cells, and that differences in the isoform α-subunit structures were responsible for their different kinase activities.

Few studies on the kinetics of IR isoform-specific internalization have been published. Yamaguchi et al. showed that in CHO cells expressing the isoforms, hIR-A displayed a 25% higher rate of ligand-stimulated internalization in comparison to hIR-B [33]. Further, work in Rat-1 fibroblasts showed that in cells expressing hIR-A, the maximum internalization reached ~65% after 10 minutes, followed by a high recycling rate of ~80% of internalized receptors after 20 minutes. In hIR-B expressing cells, the maximum internalization was ~60% and was reached within 15 minutes; however, no recycling was detectable within 30 minutes [42]. Clearly, these few data in specific cell lines warrants future research to dissect the different kinetics of internalization between the two IR isoforms.

Upon ligand-binding the IRs transduce diverse signaling pathways, which culminate in cellular functions ranging from glucose, lipid and protein metabolism to cell differentiation, proliferation and apoptosis. Insulin binding causes autophosphorylation and activation of the IR, which in turn allows the binding and activation of diverse downstream effectors. The availability and/or recruitment of specific binding partners could lead to distinct signal transductions and to the consequent activation of different pathways resulting in different biological endpoints/responses in different cell types. Up until now, only few cell types and IR isoform-specific signal transduction pathways have been investigated, especially in primary cells that express both isoforms. In the insulin-producing pancreatic β-cell, Leibiger et al. showed that the binding of insulin to IR-A or IR-B results in selective transcriptional activation of different target genes [43]. Insulin gene transcription was promoted through IR-A and the activation of PI3K class Ia/p70s6k-mediated signaling, while transcription of the glucokinase gene by signaling through IR-B PI3K class II-like activity and PKB [43]. In a subsequent study from the same group, Uhles et al. showed that isoform-specific insulin receptor signaling involves different plasma membrane domains [44]. By using tagged IR isoforms in a hamster β-cell line, they found that mutation of certain amino acids encoded by exon 11 resulted in both loss of signaling and shift in IR isoforms localization in the plasma membrane, suggesting an isoform-specific sorting to different microdomains of the plasma membrane [44]. Later, they demonstrated that spatial segregation allows simultaneous and selective signaling *via* IR-B in the same cell. They showed that in the pancreatic β-cell, insulin activated the glucokinase gene from plasma membrane-standing IR-B, while c-Fos gene activation was dependent on IR-B signaling from early endosomes [45]. In a following work, Leibiger et al. further confirmed this hypothesis by showing the co-distribution of IR-B, but not IR-A, with two proteins involved in signal transduction, PI3K-C2α and PKBα/Akt1, in the same plasma membrane microdomains [46]. In the only other system that studied the possible signaling differences between IR isoforms in primary cells, a recent work in human podocytes found that the lipid raft enzyme sphingomyelin phosphodiesterase acid-like 3b (SMPDL3b) interfered with the ability of IR-B to bind caveolin-1, thus interrupting signal transduction through this isoform. This demonstrated a mechanism *via* which sphingolipids may affect IR localization at the plasma membrane and IR signaling in an isoform-specific manner [47].

In summary, the small 12 amino acid difference between the IR isoforms is responsible for the differences in their function in studied cells where both receptors are expressed simultaneously. Thus, it will be pivotal in future research to address and consider the existence and distinction of two IR isoforms when studying insulin signaling in specific cell types.

3. Tissue and cell type IR isoform expression

The IR isoform expression is regulated in a developmental and tissue-specific manner (**Figure 2**). In human, adult tissues associated with the known metabolic effects of insulin, such as the liver, adipose tissue but also kidney, IR-B is the predominant isoform [48–51]. The IR-A isoform is highly expressed in fetal tissues—where it enhances the effects of IGF2 during embryogenesis and fetal development [52]—and in several adult tissues, such as brain [53], spleen [31], ovary [54] and testis [55]. The up-regulation of IR-A during adult life has been associated with mitogenic effects and has been described in a wide variety of cancers (reviewed in [56]). Other tissues express both isoforms in closer proportions, such as in pancreatic islets [57] and skeletal muscle [49]. Of note, IR isoform tissue distribution is generally conserved amongst mammals, with some differences, as shown in **Table 1** [31, 50, 51, 58–73].

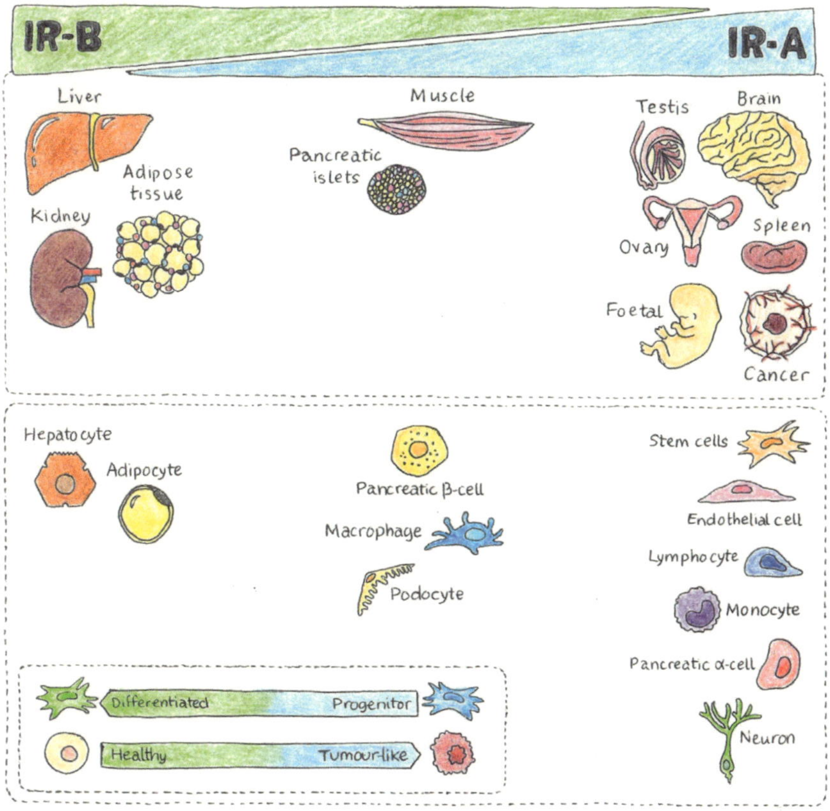

Figure 2.
IR isoform expression in tissues and cell types. IR, insulin receptor; IR-A, insulin receptor isoform A; IR-B, insulin receptor isoform B.

Because every tissue is composed of a mix of different cell types, findings regarding the expression pattern of IR isoforms cannot be extrapolated without considering the specific cell types forming the tissue. For example, analysis of liver tissue shows ~90% of IR-B expression, suggesting that hepatocytes may express exclusively IR-B. However, this tissue also contains other cell types, such endothelial cells which are known to express predominantly IR-A [70, 74], and Kupffer cells (the resident macrophages in the liver) in which IR isoform expression has not been studied. Another example is the brain, where tissue analysis shows mainly IR-A expression; however, predominant IR-B expression has been described in human astrocytes [75]. Regarding other primary cells, Muller et al. applied single-cell RT-PCR to elucidate IR isoform distribution in human pancreatic islet cells and, notably, found no expression of IR-B in isolated α-cells [69]. Mouse adipose tissue resident macrophages have been found to express both IR-A and IR-B, while mouse lymphocytes and monocytes express only a low amount of IR-B. Of note, these cells were analyzed as a bulk sample after magnetic-column cell sorting, with the possibility of low contamination of other cell types that might express IR-B [70].

IR-A is predominant in progenitor and precursor cells, whereas IR-B is more abundant in differentiated cells (**Figure 2**). Different studies reported high levels of IR-A in brown and white pre-adipocytes, osteoblast precursors, monocytes, neural progenitors and intestinal epithelial stem cells, compared with the high IR-B levels that

			Brain		Adipose tissue										Liver		Kidney		Spleen		Heart		Duodenum	
		Species			Perigonadal		Mesenteric		Retroperitoneal		Subcutaneous		Bat											
Author	Year		A	B	A	B	A	B	A	B	A	B	A	B	A	B	A	B	A	B	A	B	A	B
Besic et al.	2015	H													18	82								
Kaminska et al.	2014	H									40	60												
Mosthaf et al.	1990	H													40	60	50	50	100	0				
Seino and Bell	1989	H	100	0			70	30							15	85	40	60	100	0				
Sesti et al.	1994	H					45	55							15	85								
Vienberg et al.	2011	H									30	70												
Norgren et al.	1994	H									25	75			10	90								
Escribano et al.	2009	M													40	60								
Vienberg et al.	2011	M	95	5	22	78	25	75	38	62					5	95	5	95	95	5	60	40		
Muller et al.	2007	M																						
Moruzzi et al.[a]	2021	M	95	5	15	85					20	80	6	94	6	94	8	92	88	12	73	27	18	82
Huang et al.	1994	Mo	95	5			70	30							35	65	70	30			60	40		
Vienberg et al.	2011	P	95	5			85	15	90	10	80	20			18	92	50	50	80	20	30	70		

			Brain		Adipose tissue										Liver		Kidney		Spleen		Heart		Duodenum	
		Species			Perigonadal		Mesenteric		Retroperitoneal		Subcutaneous		Bat											
Amessou et al.	2010	R	95	5											8	92	30	70						
Serrano et al.	2005	R			40	60			50	50			40	60	0	100	30	70			50	50		
Vienberg et al.	2011	R	95	5	22	78	60	40	30	70	65	35			10	90	18	82						
Vidal et al.	1995	R			59	41									2	98					34	66		
McGrattan et al.	1998	S			29	70					29	70			20	80								
			Muscle																Pancreas		Skin		Stomach	
		Species	Hind limb		Rectus abdominis		Trapezius		EDL muscle		Soleus		GM		Vastus lateralis		White quadriceps		Islets					
Author	Year		A	B	A	B	A	B	A	B	A	B	A	B	A	B	A	B	A	B	A	B	A	B
Hribal et al.	2003	H																	50	50				
Malakar et al.	2016	H																	42	58				
Mosthaf et al.	1990	H																	80	20	90	10		
Norgren et al.	1993	H													30	70								
Sell et al.	1994	H													18	82								
Norgren et al.	1994	H			25	75																		
Malakar et al.	2016	M																	35	65				

			Muscle																Pancreas		Skin		Stomach	
		Species	Hind limb		Rectus abdominis		Trapezius		EDL muscle		Soleus		GM		Vastus lateralis		White quadriceps		Islets					
Vienberg et al.	2011	M							55	45	80	20												
Moruzzi et al.[a]	2021	M									61	39	75	25					65	35				
Huang et al.	1994	Mo													55	45							65	35
Vienberg et al.	2011	P					20	80	20	80	20	80												
Serrano et al.	2005	R									100	0					100	0	80	20				
Vienberg et al.	2011	R							90	10	90	10												
Vidal et al.	1995	R	99	1																				
McGrattan et al.	1998	S			27	73																		

BAT, brown adipose tissue; EDL muscle, extensor digitorum longus muscle; GM, gastrocnemius muscle; H, human; IR, insulin receptor; IR-A, insulin receptor isoform A; IR-B, insulin receptor isoform B; M, mouse; Mo, monkey; P, pig; R, rat; S, sheep.
[a]Control for the high-fat high-sucrose diet in that specific study.

Table 1.
IR isoform mRNA expression in humans and animal models expressed as percentage of IR-A and IR-B.

characterize their differentiated cell counterparts [70, 72, 76–79]. Some studies have reproduced this IR-A to IR-B switch favoring cell differentiation *in vitro* by overexpressing IR-B, for example in murine hemopoietic [80] and human colorectal cancer cell lines [79], or by treating HepG2 hepatoma cells with dexamethasone, which is known to maintain an adult hepatocyte phenotype [81]. These studies suggest that alternative splicing of the IR gene is a highly regulated process during differentiation and could play an important role in cell specialization.

In summary, the IR isoforms have specific tissue and cell-type distribution, and deviations from the wild-type IR-A/IR-B ratios may affect the fine-tuning of insulin signaling, disturbing metabolic and mitogenic pathways and compromising cell function.

4. Evidence of IR isoform roles using tissue-specific IR-knockout models

Insulin receptor knockout (IR-KO) mouse models have been developed to study the function of the IR, and the reconstitution of IR signaling with only one type of receptor (IR-A or IR-B) has been exploited to understanding the distinct roles of the IR isoforms. Mice with a global deletion of IR are born with normal features and with only slight growth retardation. However, shortly after birth, metabolic control rapidly deteriorates, glucose levels increase upon feeding, and insulin levels rise up to 1000-fold above normal and the animals die of diabetic ketoacidosis within 48-72 h [52, 82]. This phenotype clearly indicates that the IR is necessary for postnatal glucose homeostasis but is not essential for prenatal growth.

Using IR-KO mice, Okamoto et al. demonstrated that lethality and diabetes in IR-KO mice could be rescued by reconstitution of IR-B in three organs: liver, brain, and pancreatic β-cells [83]. However, reconstitution of IR-B in only glucose transporter type 4 (GLUT4)-expressing tissues (e.g., muscle, fat) did not rescue the phenotype [84]. Their data suggests that insulin signaling in liver, brain, and pancreatic β-cells as insulin-target tissues is sufficient to prevent diabetes. The stable expression of either IR-A or IR-B in IR-KO tissue has been used as a platform by Benito's group to study the differential role of the IR isoforms in the liver [85]. They developed adeno-associated viral vectors encoding IR-A or IR-B targeted to the liver and showed that hepatic expression of IR-A in inducible liver insulin receptor knockout (iLIRKO) mice could increase hepatic glucose utilization, thereby decreasing hyperglycemia and ameliorating the diabetic phenotype [85]. In another recent *in vivo* study, the same group explored whether overexpression of IR-A via adeno-associated viral vectors in the liver without ablation of the endogenous IR, could improve glucose homeostasis in a mouse model of high-fat diet-induced obesity [86]. Again, they observed that IR-A expression, but not IR-B expression, induced increased glucose uptake in the liver, improving insulin tolerance [86]. Of note, in both these studies a comparison of the expression levels of IR-A/B isoforms in the liver, achieved by the viral vectors, was not reported. In line with the *in vivo* findings, Nevado et al. generated immortalized neonatal hepatocyte cell lines from iLIRKO mice and reconstituted IR signaling with retroviruses encoding for human IR-A or IR-B [87]. The expression of IR-A, but not IR-B, in the iLIRKO immortalized neonatal hepatocytes restored basal glucose uptake to wild-type levels, indicating that IR-A works as a GLUT1/2-associated cotransporter to facilitate glucose uptake [87]. Consistently, Diaz-Castroverde et al. demonstrated that in iLIRKO immortalized neonatal hepatocytes, IR-A expression, but not IR-B expression, enhanced insulin signaling associated with elevated glycogen synthesis and storage [88]. It is worth noting that the primary neonatal hepatocytes *per se* might have a high IR-A/IR-B expression, which was not described. Moreover, primary hepatocytes isolated from neonatal mice were immortalized prior to the induction of IR gene knockout and reconstitution with hIR-A or hIR-B. The immortalization process may have caused an increase in IR-A expression in "wild-type cells." Thus, the restoration of IR function to "wild-type levels" mediated by IR-A could be also due to IR-A being the main isoform expressed in the immortalized neonatal hepatocytes prior to IR deletion.

To date, most of the research investigating the specific function of IR isoforms has been conducted in cell lines *in vitro*. While these experiments served for the advancement in the field, there is a clear need for more *in vivo* data. For this, a much desired mouse model would be one in which a tissue-specific IR-KO is used to reintroduce only IR-A or IR-B, which could be studied in parallel to extrapolate the gain or loss of function in IR isoform-mediated signaling in specific cell types.

5. IR isoform changes during metabolic disease

A number of *in vitro* studies have been performed to investigate the changes in IR isoform mRNA expression in response to glucose or insulin treatment [64, 66, 68]. Although it is necessary to identify possible mechanisms leading to IR splicing, the utilization of tumor-derived cells and supra-pathological amount of insulin or glucose, make it difficult to interpret these findings and reproduce them in primary cells. Moreover, the cancer cell lines used in different laboratories might have specific phenotypes regulating gene transcription machinery and the ability to modulate splicing factors in response to specific stimuli. For this reason, we have limited our discussion below to primary cells or tissues derived from humans and animal models.

In primary mammal tissues, with the tools at hand, changes in IR splicing have been studied at the transcriptional level during metabolic disease such as obesity and type 2 diabetes mellitus (T2DM), extrapolating changes to the protein level and thus signaling. During diabetes and obesity, several interesting studies addressed the possibility of splicing alteration of IR in human tissues such as muscle, liver and adipose tissue, which are accessible for sampling. Moreover, these tissues are primarily involved in insulin resistance and T2DM development, being the site of glucose handling and insulin clearance (liver), energy storage (adipose tissue) and the main site of postprandial glucose uptake (muscle).

5.1 Human evidence

In muscle, Norgren et al. found a poor correlation between IR-A mRNA and insulin-stimulated glucose utilization as well as an increase of IR-B in muscle tissue obtained from *vastus lateralis* muscle of non-insulin-dependent diabetic subjects [67]. This study was in agreement with a contemporary study conducted by Mosthaf et al., in which authors found higher IR-B expression in *vastus lateralis* muscle of subjects with insulin resistance, as compared to subjects with normal insulin sensitivity [89]. Accordingly, in a previous publication, the same authors detected predominant expression of IR-A in *gastrocnemius* of healthy subjects and both isoforms in T2DM [48]. Using a polyclonal antibody, which can differently displace radiolabeled insulin from the two IR isoforms but could not be of use for Western blot analysis (and is not commercially available), the same group corroborated their findings at the protein level and in absence of muscle fiber changes. In this work, the authors calculated an IR-A/IR-B ratio of 7:3 for control subjects and the opposite for diabetic subjects [90]. However, in another study, Benecke et al. did not find any difference in *rectus abdominis* muscle between healthy subjects compared to non-insulin-dependent T2DM patients [91]. The consensus in these studies seems to be an increase of IR-B in muscle during T2DM and T2DM development. The differences between the results can be due to the type of muscle biopsied and to the stage of T2DM. In fact, it is still unclear if different muscle fibers express different amounts of IR isoforms, which might mirror their different metabolism and glucose utilization. Thus, further work is needed to dissect these changes in muscle and the underlying mechanism using alternative methods to visualize the IR ratio *in situ*.

Contrary to muscle tissue, one study in liver suggested that hyperinsulinemia can regulate the tissue ratio of IR mRNA favoring the IR-A isoform [63]. In this work, the authors measured IR isoform mRNA levels in liver samples from individuals with or without T2DM before gastric bypass surgery and after 1.5 years follow-up. They found that IR-A expression was higher in T2DM patients prior to surgery and that the abnormal liver IR-A/IR-B ratio normalized post-surgery in patients with remission of diabetes, following a decrease in IR-A expression [63]. Despite a limited sample size, a similar trend was shown in a previous study by Moller et al. [49].

In subcutaneous adipose tissue (SAT), Kaminska et al. found an increased IR-A expression in insulin-resistant, obese and T2DM subjects (compared to controls), which was reversed by weight loss [65]. Moreover, they found a correlation between high fasting insulin and IR-A, linking these alterations to possible changes in splicing factors, which would in turn regulate IR isoform expression. However, using a polyclonal antibody which can differently displace radiolabeled insulin from the two IR isoforms (used for studies in muscle as mentioned above [90]), a previous study in human isolated adipocytes showed an increase in IR-B expression in adipocytes of non-insulin-dependent T2DM patients [92]. Notably, this small cohort of patients had similar body mass index (BMI) values and insulin levels and were on different antidiabetic medications or under dietary intervention [92].

5.2 Evidence in animal models of obesity and T2DM

In mouse as well as in other mammals, several studies have addressed the amount of IR isoform transcripts in different organs in healthy animals (see Section 3). Surprisingly, studies of the changes in IR isoform mRNA during metabolic disease, aimed to find common patterns and possible mechanisms, are scarce. The IR mRNA splicing variants were analyzed by RNA template-specific PCR (RS-PCR) in several tissues of a small group of diabetic rhesus monkeys [71]. Here, the authors showed that hyperinsulinemic monkeys had significantly higher expression of IR-A in *vastus lateralis* and *rectus abdominis* muscles compared to normoinsulinemic monkeys [71]. However, the authors did not dig into the possible mechanisms. We recently conducted a study to understand the possible splicing changes in a broad range of tissues in genetic and diet-induced mouse models of obesity and T2DM [70]. Comparing the findings to the abovementioned human studies, we found similar changes in adipose tissue, an increase in IR-A versus IR-B in all obese and diabetic mouse models, while in *soleus* and *gastrocnemius* muscles we found an increase in IR-B in the genetic models of obesity and T2DM only. Using a new method to visualize the IR mRNA isoforms *in situ* and combining it with tissue fractionation, we linked the increase of IR-A in perigonadal adipose tissue to changes in tissue architecture, rather than to a change of splice isoform in a particular cell type (i.e., adipocytes). In fact, as previously addressed, the IR isoform pattern seems to be cell-type dependent and an infiltration of immune cells (expressing mainly IR-A) in adipose tissue was the reason for these changes. The modification of tissue architecture, rather than a change of splicing at the single cell level, can also be the reason for the changes in IR isoform ratio seen in other tissues during disease. This hypothesis is further supported by a study by Vidal et al., where inducing diabetes in rats with streptozotocin showed no changes in IR mRNA ratio in liver, heart or muscle [73]. However, we have to take in consideration that rat muscle had only 1% of IR-B, the animal sample size was limited and adipose tissue was not investigated. Also, in line with this hypothesis, 48 hours of fasting in rats—which causes a significant decrease of plasma insulin—did not alter the IR isoform mRNA ratios in liver, heart, muscle and adipose tissue [73].

5.3 Myotonic dystrophy as a model of IR isoform shift

In relation to metabolic diseases, it is worth mentioning that complications of myotonic dystrophy—an autosomal genetic disease characterized by muscle loss and weakness caused by the expansion of nucleotides repeat in 3′ untranslated region of different mRNAs—has been found to alter the IR pre-mRNA splicing [93, 94]. One of the mechanisms involves the function of the CUG-BP splicing factor (acting on CUG repeats), which together with MBNL1 and other splicing factors has been shown to be pivotal for IR gene regulation [95]. In both myotonic dystrophy types 1 and 2 (DM1 and DM2), insulin resistance and decreased muscle insulin sensitivity are common. This correlates with an isoform switch from IR-B to IR-A in muscle, without changes in the total IR protein levels, and can be considered the closest model of IR splicing changes in a specific cell type *in vivo*. In this context, the diabetes medication metformin has been shown to affect the alternative splicing in DM1 patient-derived myoblast as well as in peripheral blood lymphocytes in T2DM patients, leading to the increase of IR-B expression. The increase of IR-B expression was not shared by another glucose-lowering agent, the dipeptidyl peptidase-4 (DPP-4) inhibitor sitagliptin [96]. A follow-up of this effect of metformin during T2DM treatment in other primary cells and tissue, which express both IR isoform receptors, would be of importance to understand if this could be a further mechanism explaining the effect of this drug in lowering blood glucose levels.

5.4 Summing up the evidence and the possible mechanisms

In summary, in metabolic diseases such as T2DM or obesity, limited work has been conducted in humans and animal models to uncover IR isoform changes and underlying mechanisms during disease. It seems that long-term metabolic alterations such as the ones occurring during T2DM and obesity alter the IR isoform mRNA ratio in some of the studied tissues. It seems that IR-A/IR-B ratio decreases in muscle and increases in liver and adipose tissue during hyperinsulinemic and T2DM states in humans [48, 63, 67, 89, 90, 92]. It is current consensus in the field that a higher expression of IR-A (considered to drive more mitogenic signals rather than metabolic ones) would enable this isoform to compete with IR-B for insulin, thus reducing the action of IR-B in maintaining glucose homeostasis, leading to insulin resistance. This seems to be the case during diabetes mellitus, although there could be other possible metabolic alterations due to changes in alternative splicing of other genes. Alternatively, a change in IR isoforms ratio could be interpreted as a result of changes in tissue architecture and the increase/decrease of certain cell types expressing one or the other isoforms. In fact, besides one exception, the mentioned investigations were conducted measuring IR isoform mRNA in the whole muscle, liver and adipose tissue. Architecturally, all tissues are composed of different cell types, as well as different subpopulations (heterogeneity) within a specific cell type. For example, in liver and fat, zonation has been described, in which differences in transcriptomics shows that even cells of the same kind display different phenotypes and potentially even specific IR isoform ratios [97, 98]. Thus, without experiments focusing on dissecting the mechanism behind a change in IR isoforms at single-cell resolution, it will be difficult to draw conclusion on the mechanism behind this phenomenon during metabolic disease. Future efforts are therefore required to tackle this issue more in depth to provide a common denominator for the IR changes at cell resolution, possibly taking advantage of a cell type that expresses both IR isoforms, in order to detect if changes in splicing occur.

6. Challenges and perspectives

Since the discovery of the alternative splicing of the IR in 1989 by Seino et al. [50], many studies have focused on understanding the tissue expression patterns, binding affinity, crystal structures, differential signaling and alternative routes of internalization and recycling of the IR isoforms. However, what we currently know about the IR isoforms is only a fraction of what we have not discovered yet. The reason for the two isoforms conferring an evolutionary advantage in mammals, and why other vertebrates, such as birds and fish, exist with just IR-A as well as the reasons behind the complex interactions and redundancy of insulin and IGFs systems are extremely interesting and important questions. Uncovering these aspects together with understanding why IR-A is expressed during development, in stem and cancer cells, and why progenitor cells express mainly IR-A switching their expression to IR-B upon differentiation and specialization, would help decipher the complex regulation of IR-mediated signaling upon their ligand binding. Here below, we present key points, which should be addressed in the near future, along with the tools needed in order to achieve these goals.

6.1 Shift in focus to "single cell" research

Amongst the pioneers of the IR isoform research area, Seino and Mosthaf in the '90s pinpointed the importance of determining IR isoforms splicing and their signaling at single cell level [31, 50, 99]. Until now, almost all works investigating the change in IR splice isoforms were performed using whole tissues. Thus, a key question is where/if the IR isoforms are present at the single-cell level *in vivo* in heath and disease and the possible mechanisms behind changes in their ratio. For example, in the liver, little is known about the specific expression of IR isoforms in non-parenchymal liver cells, which constitute around 20% of total cells [100]. Similar considerations apply to the brain, on which contradictory studies have been published. Garwood et al. found predominantly IR-B mRNA in cultured astrocytes isolated from human and in primary astrocytes commercially available [75]. However, this finding is difficult to reconcile with the fact that the brain tissue as a whole expresses almost only IR-A. Considering that astrocytes outnumber neurons and that the latter probably express exclusively IR-A, the expected outcome in the whole tissue following this work would be a similar expression of both isoforms. Another possible explanation would be that an IR isoform switch occurs after isolation and culture of astrocytes, or that a much lower IR mRNA is expressed in these cells compared to neurons and others cells expressing IR-A, such as endothelial cells. In contradiction, Heni et al. using another available source of human astrocytes *in vitro* found that the majority of IR mRNA in astrocytes was IR-A [101]. One single work in human brain was performed using RT-PCR/FISH to detect IR isoforms *in situ*, which in our view, lacked validation for the two IR isoforms. Nevertheless, the authors found the majority of IR mRNA as IR-B in microglia cells, and mainly IR-A in neurons, with the occasional finding of IR-B [102].

6.2 IR isoform-mediated signaling

It is common, especially in the research field of metabolic disease to talk about "classical or canonical" and "non-classical or non-canonical" insulin target tissues. The first have most commonly been liver, muscle and fat, while recently also pancreatic islets and brain have been considered. However, all cells in the body express IRs and therefore this distinction might be obsolete. The type and amount of the ligands that can bind the IR and the downstream signaling proteins involved in IR-mediated signaling (i.e., IRSs, PI3Ks, MAPKs, AKTs, etc.) are expressed in different amounts in different cell types within a tissue and this heterogeneity increases the combinatorial possibility of signaling downstream of the receptor (reviewed in [103]).

The current consensus is that an increase of IR-A, with its higher affinity for insulin and IGF2, might induce a strong proliferative signal and decrease the metabolic effect of insulin (reviewed in [56, 104]). There is strong evidence that IR-A is increased in cancer, where it exerts a proliferative and survival advantage. However, the fact that IR-A transduces a mitogenic signal in non-cancer and non-stem cells, where both isoforms are present, seems not always to be the case. In pancreatic β-cell, where both IR isoforms are present, the IR-A induces a downstream activation of insulin gene transcription and does not confer proliferative effects [43]. Of note, the pancreatic β-cell is the only primary non-cancer cell, together with kidney podocytes, from which there is evidence of IR isoform-specific signal transduction, and for which downstream pathways have been partially uncovered [43, 46, 47, 105, 106]. Moreover, cells with high prevalence of IR-A such as neurons are clearly not proliferative, showing that alteration of ligands and downstream signaling might be the key factors for the proliferative effect through IR-A.

In cells that express both IR homo-receptors simultaneously, one hypothesis would be that the two isoforms regulate different signaling pathways in the same cell as shown for pancreatic β-cells, due to spatial segregation at the membrane and different downstream binding partners. This could explain the selective insulin resistance (as shown for podocytes [47]) seen in liver or adipose tissue, where only some downstream signals of the insulin signaling pathway are blunted during disease [107, 108]. However, the selective insulin resistance in liver or fat linked to the IR isoforms still depends on the possibility that hepatocytes and adipocytes express IR-A. Moreover, if we hypothesize that of the total IR in hepatocytes or adipocytes only 10% is IR-A, then IR-A homo-receptors should be absent and IR-A would be found forming hetero-receptors with IR-B, unless some mechanism of segregation is present to preserve homo-dimer assembly.

An understudied variable that could potentially alter insulin signaling during metabolic disease is the binding of proinsulin to IR-A and its possible downstream effect. In fact, it is still not clear if this binding results in a signal transduction, or if the IR acts as a "sponge" for proinsulin resulting in a decrease in insulin binding. This aspect could play an important role during T2DM development, where the proinsulin/insulin ratio is increased in plasma [37].

In summary, much work needs to be done to understand basic questions regarding the IR isoform expression and signaling in specific cell types and during disease. However, essential tools to discriminate between the two IR isoforms are lacking and critical to address these important issues and provide breakthroughs in the field.

6.3 The need for new tools

Up until now, measuring IR isoform mRNA has been useful to investigate the isoforms at tissue level, and more recently at cellular resolution *in situ*. However, IR mRNA expression might not be linked to actual protein levels in cells and tissue [70]. One intriguing future possibility to identify the existence of IR isoforms in single cells would be to utilize single-cell RNA sequencing (RNA-Seq). However, given the low levels of IR mRNA expression and that only a few base-pairs distinguish the two isoforms, this method is still technically challenging but probably possible in the near future [109].

Pivotal to understanding the dynamics and the regulation of the equilibrium of the IR isoforms (and therefore signaling) in health and disease is to develop tools with the possibility to visualize the amount and localization of the mature isoform receptors. Up to now, attempts to develop an isoform-specific antibody for Western blotting or immunostaining have failed, probably due to the small difference between the two denatured proteins and to the fact that the 12 differential amino acids reside in a poorly accessible area of the receptor. Means to visualize the IR isoform in live cells would allow studying the binding of ligands to the IR isoforms at the cell membrane. Additionally, other small molecules such as aptamers, nucleotides oligomers that could differentially bind to the IR isoforms could conjugate with fluorescent dyes and allow the visualization of endogenous IR receptor monomers or dimers in living cells. Such visualization would allow to track the receptors *in situ* and understand more about their intracellular dynamics during health and disease. That aptamers can block IR-mediated signaling in an isoform-specific manner *in vitro* has been demonstrated [106] and shows the potential use of these molecules for IR isoform detection.

Alternatively, the results of overexpression studies can be useful in understanding the possible segregation of the IRs due to different lipid membrane requirements, and possibly signaling [110]. However, a spill over of signaling and changes in IR distribution could take place due to overexpression and the results would need to be confirmed based on the endogenous receptor.

6.4 Therapeutic potential

Let us imagine having the available methods to visualize and measure the IR at the protein level as well as the cellular distribution of IR-A/IR-B monomers, dimers and hybrids receptors. With these tools it would be possible to study which signals are transduced by the IR isoforms in a determined cell type and in response to insulin, proinsulin, IGF1 and IGF2. In this scenario, new discoveries could be used to develop targeted treatments for metabolic diseases. For example, we could screen for selective activators and inhibitors of the different IR isoforms by measuring downstream activation of selective pathways in specific healthy or diseased cells.

We have discussed the necessity of being able to understand the specific signaling cascades initiated by the different receptors upon ligand binding. The two IR isoforms could be considered as targets to selectively increase or decrease signaling pathways driven by one of the two receptors in specific cell types. Focusing on diabetes, and provided that signaling pathways downstream of IR-B are the ones modulating glucose metabolism, the generation of selective IR-B activators could be beneficial in comparison to the current insulin sensitizers or insulin analogues, which do not target either isoform specifically. On the contrary, selectively targeting IR-A, using specific antibodies or other therapeutic molecules, could be directed to treat tumor proliferation by blunting its mitogenic signaling pathways and thus hamper cell growth and survival. Newly developed insulin analogues that preferentially bind one or the other IR isoform [111] could be pivotal for improving insulin therapy, but to define this feature we would need to have tools to measure selective downstream signaling in specific cells and tissues to understand the potency and effect of such molecules. Not only peptides could be used to modulate the IR isoform activity in a selective manner, but other small molecules such as aptamers could also prove useful. One promising publication showed that these molecules can be IR isoform-specific and can facilitate or block the signaling selectively, working as allosteric regulators [112].

Another intriguing therapeutic possibility to modulate IR splice isoforms would be to use a selective splice switcher, which has recently been tested (reviewed in [113]). This would also be a better strategy to study the IR isoforms *in vitro*, since the overexpression of specific isoforms might produce a spill over of signaling cascades, as explained above.

7. Conclusions

In this chapter, we aimed to summarize the state of the art research involving the IR isoforms, especially in the area of metabolic disease. We also wanted to draw attention to how important it is to understand the full implications of having two IR isoforms. The majority of the research focused on insulin signaling refers to the IR as one receptor, without considering that there are two structurally and functionally distinct isoforms in play. In our view, future research in this field would benefit from a focus on cell type-specific IR isoform signal transduction pathways, what differences there may be between cells of the same type but different localization in a tissue, and finally, what changes occur during disease. The development of the tools needed to address these questions would pave the way for important breakthroughs in comprehending the ubiquitous, but diverse, IR signaling. Finally, these tools will be essential for the development and testing of new therapeutic strategies to counteract diseases affected by IR signaling dysfunction.

Acknowledgements

We would like to thank Ingo and Barbara Leibiger for the critical reading of this chapter and their contribution as part of the Per-Olof Berggren lab in the field of IR isoforms in pancreatic islets.

Conflicts of interest

The authors declare no conflict of interest.

Author details

Noah Moruzzi* and Francesca Lazzeri-Barcelo
The Rolf Luft Research Center for Diabetes and Endocrinology, Department of Molecular Medicine and Surgery, Karolinska Institute, Stockholm, Sweden

*Address all correspondence to: noah.moruzzi@ki.se

References

[1] Kimura KD, Tissenbaum HA, Liu Y, et al. daf-2, an insulin receptor-like gene that regulates longevity and diapause in *Caenorhabditis elegans*. Science. 1997;**277**:942-946

[2] Abbott AM, Bueno R, Pedrini MT, et al. Insulin-like growth factor I receptor gene structure. The Journal of Biological Chemistry. 1992;**267**:10759-10763

[3] Renteria ME, Gandhi NS, Vinuesa P, et al. A comparative structural bioinformatics analysis of the insulin receptor family ectodomain based on phylogenetic information. PLoS One. 2008;**3**:e3667

[4] Hernandez-Sanchez C, Mansilla A, de Pablo F, et al. Evolution of the insulin receptor family and receptor isoform expression in vertebrates. Molecular Biology and Evolution. 2008;**25**: 1043-1053

[5] Seino S, Seino M, Nishi S, et al. Structure of the human insulin receptor gene and characterization of its promoter. Proceedings of the National Academy of Sciences of the United States of America. 1989;**86**:114-118

[6] Ebina Y, Ellis L, Jarnagin K, et al. The human insulin receptor cDNA: The structural basis for hormone-activated transmembrane signalling. Cell. 1985;**40**:747-758

[7] Ullrich A, Bell JR, Chen EY, et al. Human insulin receptor and its relationship to the tyrosine kinase family of oncogenes. Nature. 1985;**313**:756-761

[8] De Meyts P, Whittaker J. Structural biology of insulin and IGF1 receptors: Implications for drug design. Nature Reviews. Drug Discovery. 2002;**1**:769-783

[9] Alarcon C, Cheatham B, Lincoln B, et al. A Kex2-related endopeptidase activity present in rat liver specifically processes the insulin proreceptor. The Biochemical Journal. 1994;**301**(Pt 1):257-265

[10] Gorden P, Arakaki R, Collier E, et al. Biosynthesis and regulation of the insulin receptor. The Yale Journal of Biology and Medicine. 1989;**62**:521-531

[11] Bravo DA, Gleason JB, Sanchez RI, et al. Accurate and efficient cleavage of the human insulin proreceptor by the human proprotein-processing protease furin. Characterization and kinetic parameters using the purified, secreted soluble protease expressed by a recombinant baculovirus. The Journal of Biological Chemistry. 1994;**269**:25830-25837

[12] Bailyes EM, Nave BT, Soos MA, et al. Insulin receptor/IGF-I receptor hybrids are widely distributed in mammalian tissues: Quantification of individual receptor species by selective immunoprecipitation and immunoblotting. The Biochemical Journal. 1997;**327**(Pt 1):209-215

[13] Yamaguchi Y, Flier JS, Benecke H, et al. Ligand-binding properties of the two isoforms of the human insulin receptor. Endocrinology. 1993;**132**:1132-1138

[14] Treadway JL, Morrison BD, Goldfine ID, et al. Assembly of insulin/insulin-like growth factor-1 hybrid receptors in vitro. The Journal of Biological Chemistry. 1989;**264**:21450-21453

[15] Frattali AL, Pessin JE. Relationship between alpha subunit ligand occupancy and beta subunit autophosphorylation in insulin/insulin-like growth

factor-1 hybrid receptors. The Journal of Biological Chemistry. 1993;**268**:7393-7400

[16] Hubbard SR, Wei L, Ellis L, et al. Crystal structure of the tyrosine kinase domain of the human insulin receptor. Nature. 1994;**372**:746-754

[17] Lou M, Garrett TP, McKern NM, et al. The first three domains of the insulin receptor differ structurally from the insulin-like growth factor 1 receptor in the regions governing ligand specificity. Proceedings of the National Academy of Sciences of the United States of America. 2006;**103**:12429-12434

[18] Croll TI, Smith BJ, Margetts MB, et al. Higher-resolution structure of the human insulin receptor ectodomain: Multi-modal inclusion of the insert domain. Structure. 2016;**24**:469-476

[19] Scapin G, Dandey VP, Zhang Z, et al. Structure of the insulin receptor-insulin complex by single-particle cryo-EM analysis. Nature. 2018;**556**:122-125

[20] Uchikawa E, Choi E, Shang G, et al. Activation mechanism of the insulin receptor revealed by cryo-EM structure of the fully liganded receptor-ligand complex. eLife. 2019;**8**:e48630

[21] Gutmann T, Schafer IB, Poojari C, et al. Cryo-EM structure of the complete and ligand-saturated insulin receptor ectodomain. The Journal of Cell Biology. 2020;**219**(1):e201907210

[22] Mynarcik DC, Yu GQ, Whittaker J. Alanine-scanning mutagenesis of a C-terminal ligand binding domain of the insulin receptor alpha subunit. The Journal of Biological Chemistry. 1996;**271**:2439-2442

[23] Whittaker J, Whittaker L. Characterization of the functional insulin binding epitopes of the full-length insulin receptor. The Journal of Biological Chemistry. 2005;**280**:20932-20936

[24] Kristensen C, Wiberg FC, Andersen AS. Specificity of insulin and insulin-like growth factor I receptors investigated using chimeric mini-receptors. Role of C-terminal of receptor alpha subunit. The Journal of Biological Chemistry. 1999;**274**:37351-37356

[25] Kristensen C, Andersen AS, Ostergaard S, et al. Functional reconstitution of insulin receptor binding site from non-binding receptor fragments. The Journal of Biological Chemistry. 2002;**277**:18340-18345

[26] Menting JG, Ward CW, Margetts MB, et al. A thermodynamic study of ligand binding to the first three domains of the human insulin receptor: Relationship between the receptor alpha-chain C-terminal peptide and the site 1 insulin mimetic peptides. Biochemistry. 2009;**48**:5492-5500

[27] Menting JG, Whittaker J, Margetts MB, et al. How insulin engages its primary binding site on the insulin receptor. Nature. 2013;**493**:241-245

[28] Hao C, Whittaker L, Whittaker J. Characterization of a second ligand binding site of the insulin receptor. Biochemical and Biophysical Research Communications. 2006;**347**:334-339

[29] Menting JG, Lawrence CF, Kong GK, et al. Structural congruency of ligand binding to the insulin and insulin/type 1 insulin-like growth factor hybrid receptors. Structure. 2015;**23**:1271-1282

[30] Whittaker J, Sorensen H, Gadsboll VL, et al. Comparison of the functional insulin binding epitopes of the A and B isoforms of the insulin receptor.

The Journal of Biological Chemistry. 2002;**277**:47380-47384

[31] Mosthaf L, Grako K, Dull TJ, et al. Functionally distinct insulin receptors generated by tissue-specific alternative splicing. The EMBO Journal. 1990; **9**:2409-2413

[32] Kellerer M, Lammers R, Ermel B, et al. Distinct alpha-subunit structures of human insulin receptor A and B variants determine differences in tyrosine kinase activities. Biochemistry. 1992;**31**:4588-4596

[33] Yamaguchi Y, Flier JS, Yokota A, et al. Functional properties of two naturally occurring isoforms of the human insulin receptor in Chinese hamster ovary cells. Endocrinology. 1991;**129**:2058-2066

[34] McClain DA. Different ligand affinities of the two human insulin receptor splice variants are reflected in parallel changes in sensitivity for insulin action. Molecular Endocrinology. 1991;**5**:734-739

[35] Frasca F, Pandini G, Scalia P, et al. Insulin receptor isoform A, a newly recognized, high-affinity insulin-like growth factor II receptor in fetal and cancer cells. Molecular and Cellular Biology. 1999;**19**:3278-3288

[36] Sacco A, Morcavallo A, Pandini G, et al. Differential signaling activation by insulin and insulin-like growth factors I and II upon binding to insulin receptor isoform A. Endocrinology. 2009;**150**:3594-3602

[37] Malaguarnera R, Sacco A, Voci C, et al. Proinsulin binds with high affinity the insulin receptor isoform A and predominantly activates the mitogenic pathway. Endocrinology. 2012;**153**:2152-2163

[38] Slaaby R, Schaffer L, Lautrup-Larsen I, et al. Hybrid receptors formed by insulin receptor (IR) and insulin-like growth factor I receptor (IGF-IR) have low insulin and high IGF-1 affinity irrespective of the IR splice variant. The Journal of Biological Chemistry. 2006;**281**:25869-25874

[39] Slaaby R. Specific insulin/IGF1 hybrid receptor activation assay reveals IGF1 as a more potent ligand than insulin. Scientific Reports. 2015;**5**:7911

[40] Benyoucef S, Surinya KH, Hadaschik D, et al. Characterization of insulin/IGF hybrid receptors: Contributions of the insulin receptor L2 and Fn1 domains and the alternatively spliced exon 11 sequence to ligand binding and receptor activation. The Biochemical Journal. 2007;**403**:603-613

[41] Pandini G, Frasca F, Mineo R, et al. Insulin/insulin-like growth factor I hybrid receptors have different biological characteristics depending on the insulin receptor isoform involved. The Journal of Biological Chemistry. 2002;**277**:39684-39695

[42] Vogt B, Carrascosa JM, Ermel B, et al. The two isotypes of the human insulin receptor (HIR-A and HIR-B) follow different internalization kinetics. Biochemical and Biophysical Research Communications. 1991;**177**:1013-1018

[43] Leibiger B, Leibiger IB, Moede T, et al. Selective insulin signaling through A and B insulin receptors regulates transcription of insulin and glucokinase genes in pancreatic beta cells. Molecular Cell. 2001;**7**:559-570

[44] Uhles S, Moede T, Leibiger B, et al. Isoform-specific insulin receptor signaling involves different plasma membrane domains. The Journal of Cell Biology. 2003;**163**:1327-1337

[45] Uhles S, Moede T, Leibiger B, et al. Selective gene activation by spatial segregation of insulin receptor B signaling. The FASEB Journal. 2007; **21**:1609-1621

[46] Leibiger B, Moede T, Uhles S, et al. Insulin-feedback via PI3K-C2alpha activated PKBalpha/Akt1 is required for glucose-stimulated insulin secretion. The FASEB Journal. 2010;**24**:1824-1837

[47] Mitrofanova A, Mallela SK, Ducasa GM, et al. SMPDL3b modulates insulin receptor signaling in diabetic kidney disease. Nature Communications. 2019;**10**:2692

[48] Mosthaf L, Vogt B, Haring HU, et al. Altered expression of insulin receptor types A and B in the skeletal muscle of non-insulin-dependent diabetes mellitus patients. Proceedings of the National Academy of Sciences of the United States of America. 1991;**88**:4728-4730

[49] Moller DE, Yokota A, Caro JF, et al. Tissue-specific expression of two alternatively spliced insulin receptor mRNAs in man. Molecular Endocrinology. 1989;**3**:1263-1269

[50] Seino S, Bell GI. Alternative splicing of human insulin receptor messenger RNA. Biochemical and Biophysical Research Communications. 1989;**159**:312-316

[51] Sesti G, Tullio AN, D'Alfonso R, et al. Tissue-specific expression of two alternatively spliced isoforms of the human insulin receptor protein. Acta Diabetologica. 1994;**31**:59-65

[52] Louvi A, Accili D, Efstratiadis A. Growth-promoting interaction of IGF-II with the insulin receptor during mouse embryonic development. Developmental Biology. 1997;**189**:33-48

[53] Pomytkin I, Costa-Nunes JP, Kasatkin V, et al. Insulin receptor in the brain: Mechanisms of activation and the role in the CNS pathology and treatment. CNS Neuroscience & Therapeutics. 2018;**24**:763-774

[54] Phy JL, Conover CA, Abbott DH, et al. Insulin and messenger ribonucleic acid expression of insulin receptor isoforms in ovarian follicles from nonhirsute ovulatory women and polycystic ovary syndrome patients. The Journal of Clinical Endocrinology and Metabolism. 2004;**89**:3561-3566

[55] Neuvians TP, Gashaw I, Hasenfus A, et al. Differential expression of IGF components and insulin receptor isoforms in human seminoma versus normal testicular tissue. Neoplasia. 2005;**7**:446-456

[56] Vella V, Milluzzo A, Scalisi NM, et al. Insulin receptor isoforms in cancer. International Journal of Molecular Sciences. 2018;**19**:3615

[57] Muller D, Huang GC, Amiel S, et al. Identification of insulin signaling elements in human beta-cells: Autocrine regulation of insulin gene expression. Diabetes. 2006;**55**:2835-2842

[58] Vienberg SG, Bouman SD, Sorensen H, et al. Receptor-isoform-selective insulin analogues give tissue-preferential effects. The Biochemical Journal. 2011;**440**:301-308

[59] Norgren S, Arner P, Luthman H. Insulin receptor ribonucleic acid levels and alternative splicing in human liver, muscle, and adipose tissue: Tissue specificity and relation to insulin action. The Journal of Clinical Endocrinology and Metabolism. 1994;**78**:757-762

[60] Escribano O, Guillen C, Nevado C, et al. Beta-cell hyperplasia induced by

hepatic insulin resistance: Role of a liver-pancreas endocrine axis through insulin receptor A isoform. Diabetes. 2009;**58**:820-828

[61] Amessou M, Tahiri K, Chauvet G, et al. Age-related changes in insulin receptor mRNA and protein expression in genetically obese Zucker rats. Diabetes & Metabolism. 2010;**36**:120-128

[62] McGrattan PD, Wylie AR, Bjourson AJ. A partial cDNA sequence of the ovine insulin receptor gene: Evidence for alternative splicing of an exon 11 region and for tissue-specific regulation of receptor isoform expression in sheep muscle, adipose tissue and liver. The Journal of Endocrinology. 1998;**159**:381-387

[63] Besic V, Shi H, Stubbs RS, et al. Aberrant liver insulin receptor isoform a expression normalises with remission of type 2 diabetes after gastric bypass surgery. PLoS One. 2015;**10**:e0119270

[64] Hribal ML, Perego L, Lovari S, et al. Chronic hyperglycemia impairs insulin secretion by affecting insulin receptor expression, splicing, and signaling in RIN beta cell line and human islets of Langerhans. The FASEB Journal. 2003;**17**:1340-1342

[65] Kaminska D, Hamalainen M, Cederberg H, et al. Adipose tissue INSR splicing in humans associates with fasting insulin level and is regulated by weight loss. Diabetologia. 2014;**57**:347-351

[66] Malakar P, Chartarifsky L, Hija A, et al. Insulin receptor alternative splicing is regulated by insulin signaling and modulates beta cell survival. Scientific Reports. 2016;**6**:31222

[67] Norgren S, Zierath J, Galuska D, et al. Differences in the ratio of RNA encoding two isoforms of the insulin receptor between control and NIDDM patients. The RNA variant without exon 11 predominates in both groups. Diabetes. 1993;**42**:675-681

[68] Sell SM, Reese D, Ossowski VM. Insulin-inducible changes in insulin receptor mRNA splice variants. The Journal of Biological Chemistry. 1994;**269**:30769-30772

[69] Muller D, Huang GC, Amiel S, et al. Gene expression heterogeneity in human islet endocrine cells in vitro: The insulin signalling cascade. Diabetologia. 2007;**50**:1239-1242

[70] Moruzzi N, Lazzeri-Barcelo F, Valladolid-Acebes I, et al. Tissue-specific expression of insulin receptor isoforms in obesity/type 2 diabetes mouse models. Journal of Cellular and Molecular Medicine. 2021;**25**:4800-4813

[71] Huang Z, Bodkin NL, Ortmeyer HK, et al. Hyperinsulinemia is associated with altered insulin receptor mRNA splicing in muscle of the spontaneously obese diabetic rhesus monkey. The Journal of Clinical Investigation. 1994;**94**:1289-1296

[72] Serrano R, Villar M, Martinez C, et al. Differential gene expression of insulin receptor isoforms A and B and insulin receptor substrates 1, 2 and 3 in rat tissues: Modulation by aging and differentiation in rat adipose tissue. Journal of Molecular Endocrinology. 2005;**34**:153-161

[73] Vidal H, Auboeuf D, Beylot M, et al. Regulation of insulin receptor mRNA splicing in rat tissues. Effect of fasting, aging, and diabetes. Diabetes. 1995;**44**:1196-1201

[74] Westermeier F, Salomon C, Farias M, et al. Insulin requires normal expression and signaling of insulin receptor A to

reverse gestational diabetes-reduced adenosine transport in human umbilical vein endothelium. The FASEB Journal. 2015;**29**:37-49

[75] Garwood CJ, Ratcliffe LE, Morgan SV, et al. Insulin and IGF1 signalling pathways in human astrocytes in vitro and in vivo; characterisation, subcellular localisation and modulation of the receptors. Molecular Brain. 2015;**8**:51

[76] Entingh AJ, Taniguchi CM, Kahn CR. Bi-directional regulation of brown fat adipogenesis by the insulin receptor. The Journal of Biological Chemistry. 2003;**278**:33377-33383

[77] Avnet S, Perut F, Salerno M, et al. Insulin receptor isoforms are differently expressed during human osteoblastogenesis. Differentiation. 2012;**83**:242-248

[78] Ziegler AN, Schneider JS, Qin M, et al. IGF-II promotes stemness of neural restricted precursors. Stem Cells. 2012;**30**:1265-1276

[79] Andres SF, Simmons JG, Mah AT, et al. Insulin receptor isoform switching in intestinal stem cells, progenitors, differentiated lineages and tumors: Evidence that IR-B limits proliferation. Journal of Cell Science. 2013;**126**:5645-5656

[80] Sciacca L, Prisco M, Wu A, et al. Signaling differences from the A and B isoforms of the insulin receptor (IR) in 32D cells in the presence or absence of IR substrate-1. Endocrinology. 2003;**144**:2650-2658

[81] Kosaki A, Webster NJ. Effect of dexamethasone on the alternative splicing of the insulin receptor mRNA and insulin action in HepG2 hepatoma cells. The Journal of Biological Chemistry. 1993;**268**:21990-21996

[82] Accili D, Drago J, Lee EJ, et al. Early neonatal death in mice homozygous for a null allele of the insulin receptor gene. Nature Genetics. 1996;**12**:106-109

[83] Okamoto H, Nakae J, Kitamura T, et al. Transgenic rescue of insulin receptor-deficient mice. The Journal of Clinical Investigation. 2004;**114**:214-223

[84] Lin HV, Accili D. Reconstitution of insulin action in muscle, white adipose tissue, and brain of insulin receptor knock-out mice fails to rescue diabetes. The Journal of Biological Chemistry. 2011;**286**:9797-9804

[85] Diaz-Castroverde S, Gomez-Hernandez A, Fernandez S, et al. Insulin receptor isoform A ameliorates long-term glucose intolerance in diabetic mice. Disease Models & Mechanisms. 2016;**9**:1271-1281

[86] Lopez-Pastor AR, Gomez-Hernandez A, Diaz-Castroverde S, et al. Liver-specific insulin receptor isoform A expression enhances hepatic glucose uptake and ameliorates liver steatosis in a mouse model of diet-induced obesity. Disease Models & Mechanisms. 2019;**12**((2):dmm036186

[87] Nevado C, Valverde AM, Benito M. Role of insulin receptor in the regulation of glucose uptake in neonatal hepatocytes. Endocrinology. 2006;**147**:3709-3718

[88] Diaz-Castroverde S, Baos S, Luque M, et al. Prevalent role of the insulin receptor isoform A in the regulation of hepatic glycogen metabolism in hepatocytes and in mice. Diabetologia. 2016;**59**:2702-2710

[89] Mosthaf L, Eriksson J, Haring HU, et al. Insulin receptor isotype expression

correlates with risk of non-insulin-dependent diabetes. Proceedings of the National Academy of Sciences of the United States of America. 1993;**90**:2633-2635

[90] Kellerer M, Sesti G, Seffer E, et al. Altered pattern of insulin receptor isotypes in skeletal muscle membranes of type 2 (non-insulin-dependent) diabetic subjects. Diabetologia. 1993;**36**:628-632

[91] Benecke H, Flier JS, Moller DE. Alternatively spliced variants of the insulin receptor protein. Expression in normal and diabetic human tissues. The Journal of Clinical Investigation. 1992;**89**:2066-2070

[92] Sesti G, Marini MA, Tullio AN, et al. Altered expression of the two naturally occurring human insulin receptor variants in isolated adipocytes of non-insulin-dependent diabetes mellitus patients. Biochemical and Biophysical Research Communications. 1991;**181**:1419-1424

[93] Savkur RS, Philips AV, Cooper TA. Aberrant regulation of insulin receptor alternative splicing is associated with insulin resistance in myotonic dystrophy. Nature Genetics. 2001;**29**:40-47

[94] Savkur RS, Philips AV, Cooper TA, et al. Insulin receptor splicing alteration in myotonic dystrophy type 2. American Journal of Human Genetics. 2004;**74**:1309-1313

[95] Sen S, Talukdar I, Liu Y, et al. Muscleblind-like 1 (Mbnl1) promotes insulin receptor exon 11 inclusion via binding to a downstream evolutionarily conserved intronic enhancer. The Journal of Biological Chemistry. 2010;**285**:25426-25437

[96] Laustriat D, Gide J, Barrault L, et al. In vitro and in vivo modulation of alternative splicing by the Biguanide Metformin. Molecular Therapy--Nucleic Acids. 2015;**4**:e262

[97] Backdahl J, Franzen L, Massier L, et al. Spatial mapping reveals human adipocyte subpopulations with distinct sensitivities to insulin. Cell Metabolism. 2021;**33**:2301

[98] Halpern KB, Shenhav R, Matcovitch-Natan O, et al. Single-cell spatial reconstruction reveals global division of labour in the mammalian liver. Nature. 2017;**542**:352-356

[99] Haring HU, Kellerer M, Mosthaf L. Modulation of insulin receptor signalling: Significance of altered receptor isoform patterns and mechanism of hyperglycaemia-induced receptor modulation. Diabetologia. 1994;**37** (Suppl. 2):S149-S154

[100] Duarte N, Coelho IC, Patarrao RS, et al. How inflammation impinges on NAFLD: A role for Kupffer cells. BioMed Research International. 2015;**2015**:984578

[101] Heni M, Hennige AM, Peter A, et al. Insulin promotes glycogen storage and cell proliferation in primary human astrocytes. PLoS One. 2011;**6**:e21594

[102] Spencer B, Rank L, Metcalf J, et al. Identification of insulin receptor splice variant B in neurons by in situ detection in human brain samples. Scientific Reports. 2018;**8**:4070

[103] Taniguchi CM, Emanuelli B, Kahn CR. Critical nodes in signalling pathways: Insights into insulin action. Nature Reviews. Molecular Cell Biology. 2006;**7**:85-96

[104] Pollak M. The insulin and insulin-like growth factor receptor family in neoplasia: An update. Nature Reviews. Cancer. 2012;**12**:159-169

[105] Leibiger IB, Leibiger B, Berggren PO. Insulin feedback action on pancreatic beta-cell function. FEBS Letters. 2002;**532**:1-6

[106] Leibiger B, Moede T, Paschen M, et al. PI3K-C2alpha knockdown results in rerouting of insulin signaling and pancreatic beta cell proliferation. Cell Reports. 2015;**13**:15-22

[107] Brown MS, Goldstein JL. Selective versus total insulin resistance: A pathogenic paradox. Cell Metabolism. 2008;**7**:95-96

[108] Tan SX, Fisher-Wellman KH, Fazakerley DJ, et al. Selective insulin resistance in adipocytes. The Journal of Biological Chemistry. 2015;**290**:11337-11348

[109] Arzalluz-Luque A, Conesa A. Single-cell RNAseq for the study of isoforms-how is that possible? Genome Biology. 2018;**19**:110

[110] Gerdes JM, Christou-Savina S, Xiong Y, et al. Ciliary dysfunction impairs beta-cell insulin secretion and promotes development of type 2 diabetes in rodents. Nature Communications. 2014;**5**:5308

[111] Chrudinova M, Zakova L, Marek A, et al. A versatile insulin analog with high potency for both insulin and insulin-like growth factor 1 receptors: Structural implications for receptor binding. The Journal of Biological Chemistry. 2018;**293**:16818-16829

[112] Yunn NO, Koh A, Han S, et al. Agonistic aptamer to the insulin receptor leads to biased signaling and functional selectivity through allosteric modulation. Nucleic Acids Research. 2015;**43**:7688-7701

[113] Havens MA, Hastings ML. Splice-switching antisense oligonucleotides as therapeutic drugs. Nucleic Acids Research. 2016;**44**:6549-6563

Chapter 3

Molecular Mechanisms Involved in Insulin Resistance: Recent Updates and Future Challenges

Atamjit Singh, Nikhita Ghai and Preet Mohinder Singh Bedi

Abstract

Insulin resistance (IR) is a condition in which insulin-mediated regulation of glucose metabolism in body tissues (primarily liver, adipose tissue and skeletal muscle) becomes disrupted. IR is a characteristic marker of type 2 diabetes and cardiovascular diseases. IR is generally associated with metabolic abnormalities, including hyperinsulinemia, impaired glucose homeostasis, hyperlipidemia and obesity. IR can arise from pathological, genetic and environmental factors or from a combination of these factors. Studies conducted in recent decades showcase the important role of adipose tissue in the development of IR via release of lipids and different circulating factors. These extracellular factors influence the intracellular levels of intermediates including ceramide and various lipids that influence the cell responsiveness to insulin. These intermediates are suggested to promote IR via inhibition of one or more components of insulin signaling pathway (e.g., insulin receptor, insulin receptor substrate proteins). This chapter will shed light on various molecular mechanisms and factors contributing to IR, which will help the researchers to design potential therapeutic strategies and interventions for efficiently managing IR and its related disorders.

Keywords: insulin, insulin receptor, insulin resistance, glucose uptake, glucose metabolism

1. Introduction

Following a meal, pancreatic β-cells produce insulin in response to increasing blood glucose and other metabolite levels for regulating systemic glucose homeostasis. Tissue insulin sensitivity, which characterizes the ability of a given concentration of insulin to correct blood glucose levels, is the driving force behind this homeostasis. Multiple processes in several organs are involved in this typically well-regulated homeostatic mechanism, including decreased glucose output from the liver (hepatic glucose output), increased glucose uptake into skeletal muscle and adipose tissue (where glucose is stored as glycogen), suppression of free fatty acid (FFA) release from adipocytes (suppression of lipolysis), and increased lipid accumulation in the liver and adipocytes. A sophisticated insulin-dependent signal transduction cascade controls these metabolic processes. Insulin resistance (IR) is defined as decreased insulin-stimulated glucose uptake into muscle and adipocytes and faulty insulin regulation of hepatic glucose production in patients with type 2 diabetes (T2D) and in many subjects affected by other conditions characterized by insulin resistance, such as obesity and polycystic ovary syndrome. The term insulin resistance was first coined to explain the considerable variability in the insulin dose necessary to lower high glucose levels in people with T2D, and then to characterize the magnitude of change in blood glucose level when a given amount of insulin and glucose was administered. The "defined quantity of insulin" is crucial because people with insulin resistance often have hyperinsulinemia, a condition in which insulin levels in the blood are higher than normal relative to the amount of blood glucose concentration under both fasting and fed conditions; this hyperinsulinemia compensates for IR in peripheral tissues to bring blood glucose levels back to normal [1].

When pancreas fails to supply excess insulin in humans with insulin resistance, a major defect in whole-body glucose homeostasis occurs, resulting in hyperglycemia and glucose intolerance (the latter including impaired fasting glucose and impaired glucose tolerance), which are the defining features of T2D. It is worth noting that, somewhat counterintuitively, patients with T2D frequently maintain "relative hyperinsulinemia" until the condition is at an advanced stage. IR is defined by insulin's inability to induce glucose uptake into muscle and adipose cells due to a failure of the glucose transport mechanism mediated, at the molecular level, by glucose transporter type 4 (GLUT4) in those tissues. Furthermore, one of the hallmarks of IR is the inability to decrease hepatic glucose production, which is mostly due to a persistent increase in hepatic gluconeogenesis. IR has been linked to a variety of diseases. Indeed, IR represents a risk factor for various conditions, such as metabolic disorders (including T2D and obesity), heart disease, liver diseases (e.g., non-alcoholic fatty liver disease and non-alcoholic steatohepatitis), cancer, neurodegenerative diseases and frailty [2–4]. Despite the fact that IR is inextricably linked to T2D, an important factor involved in T2D pathophysiology is represented by the pancreas' incapacity to function properly to compensate for the significant rise in blood glucose levels by secreting enough insulin to meet the increasing demand and help get blood glucose levels back to normal. IR is a key risk factor for T2D, yet it is not commonly recognized or treated in people without diabetes. The main reason for this phenomenon is that many people with insulin resistance do not have abnormal blood glucose levels. Therefore, diagnosis of IR is based on measuring insulin levels, which is not commonly done in clinical practice. Furthermore, only a small fraction of subjects with IR develop T2D, which is likely due to a propensity to β-cell failure in these subjects. There are no procedures to identify this susceptible subpopulation at this time. Individuals with IR are predisposed to significant disorders linked to T2D, including retinopathy, neuropathy and kidney disease, even if they do not have T2D [5]. In this chapter, the association between the early possible causes of IR is first discussed. Obesity is common in people with IR, but it is unclear whether concomitant hyperinsulinemia contributes to obesity development or whether it is a consequence of obesity-associated IR. We then look at how different metabolic tissues, such as muscle, adipose tissue, and the liver, communicate with one another. The mechanisms of impaired insulin signaling and the role of abnormal GLUT4 trafficking in the development of IR are also discussed. Extracellular factors that may contribute to IR are postulated. This discussion is then followed by a discussion of various intracellular molecular factors that contribute to IR. These factors have been considered as involved in processes that lead to IR. There are several ways for determining insulin action. Many laboratories have lately resorted to employing surrogate markers of insulin sensitivity and IR [6].

The "traditional" definition of IR is a condition in which blood glucose levels are abnormally high and insulin concentration needed to maintain glucose homeostasis is greater than predicted [7, 8].

2. Pathway to insulin resistance

Despite years of research, there is still a lot of uncertainty about the causative and temporal link between obesity, hyperinsulinemia, and IR. The proximal and distal parts of the insulin signaling system, which governs metabolism, can be arbitrarily partitioned. The classical components—which comprise the insulin receptor, insulin receptor substrate (IRS) proteins, phosphoinositide 3-kinase (PI3K) and AKT-constitute the proximal segment of the insulin signaling system. A common trait of the proximal components is their sparseness, which means that just a little part of each element is necessary to elicit a physiological signal. This guarantees signal amplification across the network. The proximal portion is also susceptible to very complex feedforward and feedback control, and is incorporated into a broader network that is dynamically regulated by combinatorial signaling inputs. The AKT substrates that are intimately related to the many physiological activities of insulin and are typically specialized to a particular cell type are referred to as the "distal segment" of the insulin signaling pathway. The distal elements are generally phosphorylated, which is a common trait. Insulin signaling begins with the hormone binding to its surface receptor, followed by activation of the receptor tyrosine kinase and tyrosine phosphorylation. IRS proteins are phosphorylated, causing them to create a signaling complex, which contains proteins with Src homology domains such as PI3K. As a result, phosphatidylinositol (3,4,5)-trisphosphate [PtdIns(3,4,5)P3 or PIP3] is produced. Serine/threonine (Ser/Thr) protein kinases like PDK1 and AKT, for example, are recruited to the inner leaflet of the plasma membrane. AKT is phosphorylated by PDK1 at one of its phosphorylation sites. Partially phosphorylated AKT activates mTORC2, while phosphorylation of AKT specifically at Ser473 results in complete AKT activation. Thus, AKT is a critical node in the insulin signaling pathway. AKT performs a variety of biological roles and is involved in the majority, if not all, of physiological metabolic processes. The Rab GTPase-Activating Protein (GAP) is an AKT substrate, which activates TBC1D4 (TBC1 Domain Family Member 4), a protein that regulates GLUT4 trafficking within the plasma membrane. The activation of glucose transport by insulin is the key mechanism that is disrupted in insulin-resistant muscle and fat cells. The GLUT4 is a facilitative glucose transporter, which is found in skeletal muscle, heart, adipocytes, and insulin-responsive neurons; it regulates muscle/fat glucose transfer. Unlike other transporters (like GLUT1), GLUT4 has a set of specific trafficking cues that let it migrate from endosomes and the trans-Golgi network (TGN) to a special intracellular population of vesicles known as "GLUT4 storage vesicles" (GSVs) [9–11]. GSVs act as a distinct controlled exocytic compartment that distributes GLUT4 to the cell surface in response to insulin and serves as a storage depot assuring low rates of glucose absorption in the fasting state. Although exercise increases GLUT4 translocation in muscle cells, it does so through a different mechanism than that regulated by insulin. AKT plays a critical role in the insulin-regulated GLUT4 translocation [12, 13]. These characteristics typically coexist, and there is strong evidence that each can cause the other two branches of the triad to emerge: obesity, hyperinsulinemia, and IR are caused by overnutrition in humans and animals; in humans, IR and obesity may also be caused by continuous insulin administration or by genetic factors; in addition, IR in humans may be caused by pharmacological interventions resulting in hyperinsulinemia [14, 15].

3. The trio-axis of obesity-hyperinsulinemia-insulin resistance

Obesity and IR are two topics that come up frequently. The long period during which obesity, IR and hyperinsulinemia develop, makes the determination of causative links between these conditions (which usually coexist in most persons with T2D at the time of diagnosis) particularly difficult. Obesity is common in people with IR, although it is unclear whether simultaneous hyperinsulinemia plays a role in obesity development or it is predominantly a result of obesity-dependent IR [16]. The study of first-degree relatives of people with T2D who only show some of these traits has shown to be one of the most effective strategies for addressing some unanswered questions in humans. As a result, a trait seen in relatives is more likely to appear early in the course of the disease. It has been found that these subjects can have considerable IR in skeletal muscle and liver (and possibly fat), along with modest hyperinsulinemia, even if they are not obese or glucose-intolerant [15, 17, 18]. Individuals who are lean and glucose-tolerant but exhibit IR have been identified in larger cross-sectional studies [19]. In these instances, obesity is unlikely to be the primary cause of tissue IR. However, the term "obesity" is defined differently depending on race and genetic background, and it should therefore used with caution. Body mass index may be more important in determining the risk of IR. Body weight, in general, and visceral fat (but not subcutaneous fat), in particular, should be considered for evaluation [20].

First-degree relatives of people with T2D had greater levels of circulating FFAs and intramuscular lipids than healthy control subjects [21], suggesting that intramyocellular lipid content represents an early abnormality in the pathogenesis of insulin resistance and that it may contribute to the impaired glucose uptake in skeletal muscle of insulin-resistant subjects to a greater extent than overall adiposity. This is in line with severe IR observed in patients with lipodystrophy syndromes, which are a heterogeneous group of diseases characterized by selective absence of adipose tissue, loss of functional adipocytes, ectopic steatosis, and severe dyslipidemia and IR [22, 23]. On the other hand, individuals with moderate or severe obesity can be "metabolically healthy" [24]. While it appears acceptable, based on this research, to conclude that obesity is not a risk factor essential for the development of IR, it is vital to highlight that the majority of subjects with IR are obese. As we will discuss later in the text, the amount and location of adiposity required to create IR varies greatly between subjects.

4. Insulin resistance and hyperinsulinemia

Defining the temporal link between hyperinsulinemia and IR is difficult since, as far as we know, IR does not exist in the absence of hyperinsulinemia in humans, and vice versa. Hyperinsulinemia can produce obesity and IR in humans, as evidenced by trials in which insulin is administered to induce hyperinsulinemia in otherwise healthy individuals or as it occurs naturally in people with insulinomas [25, 26]. Transgenic expression of multiple copies of the normal insulin gene causes hyperinsulinemia in mice, resulting in IR and glucose intolerance [27]. Inhibition of insulin secretion has also been shown to improve insulin sensitivity and to decrease body weight in rodents [28–30]. In mice, deletion of one copy of the insulin gene resulted in a reduction of the Western diet-induced hyperinsulinemia and in an improvement of insulin sensitivity [31]. Overall, the hypotheses that hyperinsulinemia causes IR and promotes obesity, or that IR associated with obesity causes hyperinsulinemia, both remain acceptable for the initial events involved in T2D pathophysiology. In actuality, IR and hyperinsulinemia coexist and lead to T2D in almost all cases [32]. Several data suggest a concept in which hyperinsulinemia is responsible for, or at least partly contributes to, many of the negative effects of IR; this implies that IR is a state in which many of the insulin actions are preserved, a condition known as "selective IR" [33–35]. This was first observed in the liver, where increased insulin levels are unable to decrease hepatic glucose output in people with T2D, although lipogenesis (a canonical insulin action in the liver) remains elevated [36, 37]. One explanation for this selectivity is that insulin signaling pathway in the liver splits into two arms, with IR affecting only the arm regulating hepatic gluconeogenesis but not the arm regulating lipid metabolism. Hepatic de novo lipogenesis is essentially a cell-autonomous phenomenon, whereas cell-nonautonomous suppression of hepatic glucose production by insulin depends upon the insulin-mediated decrease of adipocyte lipolysis and circulating FFAs [38]. There has also been evidence of selective IR in muscle and adipose tissue. Those insulin-regulated activities which are not affected by IR—such as lipogenesis, protein synthesis, or transcriptional control mediated by FOXO proteins—are hyperactivated in the context of hyperinsulinemia and are likely to worsen IR or its consequences [33, 34, 39, 40].

5. Heterogeneity in the development of insulin resistance and progression of metabolic disease and T2D

T2D patients are divided into different phenotypic clusters based on their symptoms and clinical features. Individuals in one of these groups share phenotypic traits. As a result, performing a comprehensive analysis of these groups will be of great importance in clinical settings. Phenotype data analysis and combination of phenotype data with genetic data are essential to gain a better understanding of the variability in the development and presentation of IR in humans [10, 11, 41].

6. Tissue-specific progression to insulin resistance

The appearance of IR occurs in various tissues in a specific order. The development of IR in several tissues—including skeletal muscle, liver, and adipose tissue—is a hallmark of fully developed T2D in humans [18, 19, 39, 40, 42]. Evidence shows a hierarchical progression of IR in skeletal muscle, liver and adipose tissue, whereby IR develops in one tissue and then spreads to other tissues via systemic circulating components. For example, IR in the liver and adipose tissue appears to occur prior to IR in muscle in C57Bl/6 mice fed a high-fat diet [43–46]. An equivalent pattern in humans is unlikely, since first-degree relatives of persons with T2D who are in the early stages of the disease already have IR in both muscle and liver (and possibly fat) [47]. Since insulin sensitivity in humans is often measured as whole-body glucose consumption (to which adipose tissue contributes only to a small extent), the temporal development of IR in adipose tissue in humans is less obvious. Interestingly, multiple investigations show that insulin modulates hepatic glucose production via reducing adipocyte lipolysis in a non-cell-autonomous manner [45]. Given these findings, it is reasonable to believe that adipose tissue IR is a precursor to metabolic disease and T2D. However, there is a clear distinction between insulin action on the liver and insulin action on muscle: even in people with T2D, the defect in insulin sensitivity in the liver can be almost completely overcome by sufficiently high levels of insulin, whereas muscle (and fat) insulin sensitivity defects persist at higher insulin concentrations [40, 48, 49]. This indicates that the processes that cause IR in muscle and liver are distinct.

Tissue-specific insulin receptor gene knockouts in mice have provided persuasive evidence that IR in a particular tissue can at least spread to other organs. Experimenting with a specific deficiency in insulin action in muscle, fat, or liver has resulted in the spread of IR to other tissues in a number of cases [50]. However, depending on the tissue that is first targeted and/or in which a specific gene deletion occurs, the mechanism of inter-tissue communication varies. The deletion of GLUT4, which is essential for glucose uptake in adipose tissue and skeletal muscle, is one of the best examples of this inter-tissue communication. In mice, deletion of GLUT4 resulted in IR not only in the tissue from which the transporter was removed, but also in all metabolic tissues, including the liver. Surprisingly, normalization of blood glucose levels reverses IR in the liver and adipose tissue in muscle-specific Glut4 gene-knockout mice. This shows that glucotoxicity generated IR in this animal model, which is not the case in many other IR models, including the Western diet-fed C57BL/6J mice, which do not show considerable hyperglycemia [48–51]. As a result, while these animal studies have been useful in uncovering mechanisms of IR in specific tissues, their clinical applicability is less evident because complete deletion of a gene preferentially in one tissue does not occur in humans. Nonetheless, these experiments have provided persuasive evidence that metabolic or signaling changes in one tissue can have systemic effects by influencing insulin activity in other organs, a phenomenon that has been well-validated by clinical findings [50, 51].

7. Impaired insulin signaling in insulin resistance

Over the past 40 years, much research has resulted in a precise understanding of the insulin signaling system, which mediates the insulin's physiological activities. One popular theory is that IR is caused by a defect in one or more of these signaling components. Another viewpoint is that IR is only caused by a shift in metabolic flux. For example, since the 1960s fatty acids have been proven to impede cells' ability to utilize carbohydrate by allosterically modifying crucial rate-limiting steps in carbohydrate metabolic pathways. Several pieces of evidence, however, refute this claim. IR can be seen in cells or tissues long after the animal tissues have been removed, implying that changes that contribute to IR are long-lasting and cannot be explained by the acute action of a systemic factor. Fatty acids decrease the insulin-dependent translocation of GLUT4 to the plasma membrane and limit glucose uptake, there is no indication that this inhibition is caused by an allosteric change of GLUT4. Finally, IR can persist even after significant changes in dietary intake and after changes in metabolic state induced by pharmacological interventions. Thus, based on this information, it is reasonable to believe that IR is caused by an alteration in insulin signaling, although the exact location of the defect in the insulin signaling pathway remains unknown. Many essential components of the insulin signaling system have been identified. These components are divided into two parts: (i) the proximal part, which represents the core canonical signaling pathway, which includes the insulin receptor, IRS, PI3K and AKT; and (ii) the distal part, which includes TBC1D4, GSK3 (glycogen synthase kinase-3) and PDE3B (phosphodiesterase 3B). IR has been linked to defects in proximal insulin signaling system, that are associated with cellular stress. Many of the intracellular stressors discussed in the next sections activate a variety of intracellular Ser/Thr kinases, including novel PKCs (protein kinase C), JNK (c-Jun amino-terminal kinase), mTOR (mammalian target of rapamycin)and S6 kinase, which phosphorylate either the insulin receptor or the insulin receptor-related protein (INSRR). This could be a negative-feedback route that inhibits insulin signaling, according to the theory. However, as it will be discussed later, mounting evidence suggests that proximal insulin signaling system is unaffected in IR, implying that IR is caused by abnormalities in distal components of the insulin signaling network [52–54].

8. Insulin resistance and insulin signaling at the proximal level

The current focus on proximal insulin signaling abnormalities as a cause of IR stems from research into rare, monogenic severe types of IR that were discovered to be caused by mutations in the insulin receptor gene or by the development of insulin receptor blocking antibodies. Because of the superficial parallels between these rare conditions and T2D, it is reasonable to conclude that both diseases are caused by abnormalities in insulin receptor function, with the degree of receptor failure varying only slightly. Despite early enthusiasm for this theory, subsequent research found that IR in most forms of T2D was caused by neither impaired insulin receptor activity nor changes in the expression or quantity of insulin receptors. Insulin-binding experiments in rat adipocytes found that only 2.4% of total insulin receptors are required for a full biological response, implying that metabolic cells like muscle, fat and liver cells have an abundance of insulin receptors; this finding became known as the "spare insulin receptor" hypothesis. Insulin-mediated glucose uptake is reduced in insulin-resistant skeletal muscle cells and adipocytes. Since a slight decrease in the number of insulin receptors could only diminish insulin sensitivity and not the maximal insulin response [54–58]. While some studies contradict the "spare insulin receptor" hypothesis, recent genetic studies in mice support the idea that insulin signaling is preserved when the number of insulin receptors is reduced: mice with heterozygous loss of the insulin receptor had normal glucose and insulin tolerance and no impairment in AKT signaling in muscle or adipose tissue [59–62].

The concept of spare insulin receptors shifted focus to a "postreceptor defect", which is represented by defects in signaling downstream intermediates of the insulin receptor as the cause of IR [57, 58, 63]. Loss-of-function mutations in a number of signaling genes—including TBC1D4, AKT2, and IRS1 in humans—have been linked to severe forms of IR and T2D; moreover, cancer treatments that block PI3K or AKT have been linked to IR and T2D in humans. IR is caused in mice by targeted deletion of these genes. In addition, IR results in reduction of skeletal muscle AKT phosphorylation in response to insulin stimulation [34, 64, 65].

Given evidence of "spareness" for IRS, PI3K and AKT, the possibility that abnormalities in proximal insulin signaling might be responsible for IR has to be questioned, in the same way that the "spare receptor" theory has to be questioned. Homozygous deletion of AKT2, the most prevalent AKT gene isoform, resulted in a 90% reduction in insulin-stimulated AKT phosphorylation, but with no discernible defect in phosphorylation of the AKT substrate, or protein synthesis in response to insulin.

In this situation, there was a tiny quantity of AKT1 expression that was not influenced by the gene deletion and was enough to deliver a completely functional message as response to insulin [66, 67]. Similarly, whereas AKT2 accounts for 85% of total AKT in the liver, its ablation does not result in significant glucose intolerance because the remaining AKT1 compensates for this defect [68]. The insulin dose-response curve in adipocytes, where the curve for AKT phosphorylation is "shifted to the right" compared to that for AKT substrate phosphorylation or insulin action, indicates that partial phosphorylation of AKT is sufficient for maximal biological responses, providing additional evidence for "spareness" in proximal insulin signaling network. At "normal" insulin concentrations, phosphorylation of AKT substrates requires only 1% of the entire AKT pool to be activated [69–71]. Furthermore, AKT phosphorylation is reduced in muscle from T2D patients, while downstream substrate phosphorylation is unaffected. Importantly, studies in animals fed a Western diet have indicated that IR begins before any detectable insulin signaling defect. Only 42 days of Western diet feeding resulted in reduced insulin-stimulated AKT phosphorylation, but TBC1D4 phosphorylation remained normal. As a result, minor changes in phosphorylation of proximal insulin signaling components may result in insulin sensitivity, but they are unlikely to result in a reduction in the maximal physiologic response [53].

Thus, how can the predominance of abnormalities in proximal insulin signaling components observed in diverse IR models, such as lower AKT phosphorylation, be reconciled? It is possible that these defects are a result of defective glucose metabolism rather than the cause. This could be a direct effect secondary to compensatory hyperinsulinemia, a typical hallmark of IR (since persistent hyperinsulinemia can lead to degradation of proximal insulin signaling components); alternatively, it may be a cell-autonomous effect due to a reduction in AKT phosphorylation as a result of defective glycolysis. Many studies used insulin-stimulated AKT phosphorylation in mice (sometimes in response to a maximal, pharmacological dosage of insulin) as an indicator of insulin sensitivity [72–75].

However, under physiological settings such as the response to a meal (with minimal insulin release), AKT phosphorylation is barely detectable, due to the non-linearity between AKT phosphorylation and phosphorylation of its substrates. As a result, when evaluating the physiological importance of insulin signaling, it is critical to look at the phosphorylation of a variety of AKT substrates to determine if there is a major deficiency in "AKT activity" in vivo. These findings suggest that a minor impairment in proximal insulin signaling network is unlikely to account for the significant reduction in insulin-stimulated glucose uptake observed in patients with T2D. Furthermore, these findings underline that lower AKT2 phosphorylation should not be used as a direct marker or even as a proxy measure of IR [71].

Negative feedback loops originating from Ser/Thr kinases that phosphorylate and limit the action of IRS proteins have also been proposed as a cause of IR. This theory is refuted by a number of studies. Since Platelet-derived growth factor (PDGF) by-passes these proteins to activate glucose uptake, mice bred to overexpress PDGF receptor (PDGFR) in muscle presented an ideal model to explore whether deficiencies in insulin receptor or IRS were implicated in experimental IR. In these mice, PDGF treatment resulted in increased glucose uptake in muscle [76]. Notably, when PDGFR transgenic rats were fed a Western diet, muscle glucose uptake in response to PDGF was decreased to the same degree as insulin-mediated uptake. This refutes a role for inhibitory Ser/Thr phosphorylation of the insulin receptor or IRS as a cause of IR, indicating that the deficiency in glucose uptake or IR does not involve the insulin receptor or IRS [8, 53, 54, 77, 78].

Furthermore, in mice, targeted mutation of one of the major putative inhibitory sites in IRS1 (Ser307), deletion of potential mediators of IR, such as PKC (which is reported to phosphorylate insulin receptor), and pharmacological blockade of key negative feedback pathways, such as mTOR (which is activated by insulin signaling and inhibits signaling by phosphorylating IRS through a negative feedback mechanism) [78–81].

Finally, investigations in humans with IR or T2D revealed that insulin-stimulated muscle glucose uptake is reduced by 50–100% even at maximum insulin dosages [82–85], with no change or reduction in AKT phosphorylation [86–88]. Only a few of these studies addressed the mechanism of AKT substrate phosphorylation in depth, and those that did found no deficiency or poorly linked with IR. These findings support the theory that the proximal insulin signaling network in human tissues has enough "spareness" to overcome even a moderate deficiency in AKT phosphorylation [87–89], and that lowered AKT phosphorylation is adequate to ensure a normal signal transduction. As previously stated, faulty proximal insulin signaling is most likely a result of IR rather than a cause of IR [90].

9. GLUT4 and insulin resistance

Insulin stimulates the transfer of intracellular GLUT4 storage vesicles to the cell surface, resulting in glucose uptake in skeletal muscle cells and adipocytes (**Figure 1**) [91–94]. Insulin-dependent GLUT4 translocation has been linked to IR in both skeletal muscle and adipose tissue. This decrease in GLUT4 availability at the plasma membrane causes a reduced glucose uptake, which can lead to other IR-related consequences like reduced AKT phosphorylation, protein synthesis defects, and increased lipolysis [72, 95, 96]. GLUT4 does not show spareness, unlike proximal insulin signaling components such as IRS1 and AKT. The fact that heterozygous GLUT4 gene-knockout mice acquire metabolic disease exemplifies this concept [97].

However, while GLUT4 levels are lowered by 50% in human adipose tissue from patients with T2D, such levels remain unaltered in skeletal muscle, implying that GLUT4 levels cannot explain IR development in skeletal muscle [98].

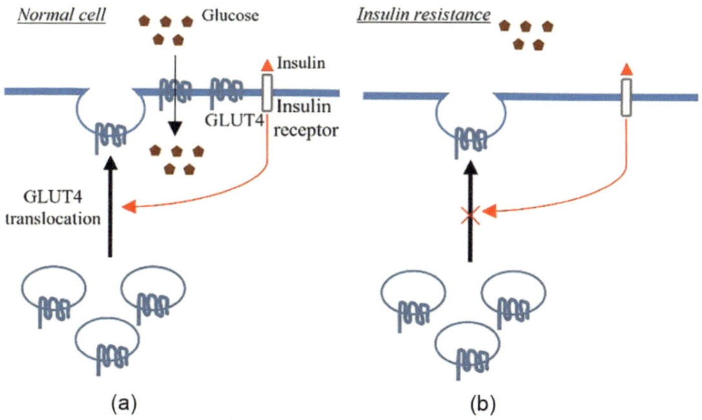

Figure 1.
Translocation of glucose transporter type 4 (GLUT4) from GLUT4 storage vesicles (GSVs) to the plasma membrane of normal adipocytes and skeletal muscle cells (a). This process is altered in conditions characterized by insulin resistance (b).

Despite normal GLUT4 levels, insulin-stimulated GLUT4 translocation to the cell surface in skeletal muscle is faulty in both individuals with T2D [92] and in several rodent models of IR [99, 100]. Importantly, while exercise-modulated GLUT4 translocation to the cell surface is unaffected [101], the impairment in muscle GLUT4 trafficking in T2D is insulin signaling-specific. Insulin and exercise both cause GLUT4 translocation to the cell surface from discrete intracellular compartments [102].

The ultimate defect that defines IR is the impaired GLUT4 translocation to the plasma membrane. However, it is unknown how the numerous potential intracellular IR mediators mentioned later affect GLUT4 trafficking. Three options are discussed here. First, GLUT4 translocation requires that GLUT4 is localized in the appropriate intracellular compartment, the so-called GLUT4 storage vesicles (GSVs); GLUT4 targeting to GLUT4 GSVs has been hypothesized to be altered in IR [91, 100]. However, whereas this would likely result in GLUT4 degradation, GLUT4 levels in skeletal muscle from patients with IR remain unaffected. Second, given the importance of protein phosphorylation in insulin action [101–104], it is possible that the defect is caused by a distal component of the insulin-regulated phosphorylation network such as TBC1D4, which regulates GLUT4 trafficking, although there is no convincing evidence for defective TBC1D4 phosphorylation in IR [105]. TBC1D4 is unlikely to be the only AKT target causing GLUT4 translocation, as cells lacking TBC1D4 still have some insulin-sensitive glucose transport [106]. Recent phosphoproteomics studies have revealed the existence of a wide range of insulin-responsive phosphoproteins in metabolic cells, allowing for the identification of insulin signaling targets in the distal part of the insulin signaling pathway that may be involved in the development of IR [104]. Indeed, IR is associated with massive alterations in the architecture of the entire insulin signaling pathway, according to examination of muscle cells from T2D patients [107]. Finally, a direct alteration of GLUT4 or a defect in a yet undiscovered protein that interacts with GLUT4 could cause the abnormalities in GLUT4 trafficking. This could include carbonylation and oxidation-induced inactivation of GLUT4, which have been observed in humans as a response to short-term overnutrition [108]. Protein carbonylation is linked to H_2O_2 production, lipid peroxidation and IR, suggesting a link between such molecular processes and the development of IR [109].

10. Adipose tissue and insulin resistance

While IR is regularly seen in lean first-degree relatives of patients with T2D, it is also found in many lean "healthy" individuals, suggesting that IR is more common than previously thought. In this regard, dietary habits, physical activity level and genetics are important factors that can significantly contribute to IR. Adipose tissue makes a significant contribution to the development of IR. Limitations in peripheral adipose tissue storage capacity and expansion in response to over nutrition (as it occurs in overweight and obesity) lead to increased circulating lipids, subsequent lipid accumulation in non-adipose tissues (ectopic lipid in liver, skeletal muscle, heart, and pancreas) and development of lipid-induced IR and metabolic derangements [110, 111]. Because of this, and since there is a clear link between IR and increased adipose tissue mass, we will discuss the role of adipose tissue mass and lipotoxicity as significant drivers of IR, as well as the emerging mechanisms by which adipocytes contribute to systemic IR.

10.1 Adipose tissue dysfunction

IR in adipocytes could be the first step in the progression of adipose tissue dysfunction, similar to IR in muscle and liver. In adipocytes from first-degree relatives of patients with T2D, there is a low expression of markers of insulin sensitivity such as GLUT4 and adiponectin (a crucial systemic insulin-sensitizing adipokine produced by adipose tissue), supporting this theory [112]. Furthermore, adipocyte hypertrophy (increase in adipocyte size) appears to precede T2D onset in Pima Indians, a group of Native Americans with a high incidence of IR and T2D [113]. Additionally, mouse models with adipose-specific IR also have IR in their muscle and liver. Notably, IR in the muscle of adipose-specific Glut4 gene-knockout mice was only present in vivo but not when muscles were isolated and assessed in vitro, implying a role for systemic factors (which did not include circulating FFAs or inflammatory cytokines) in the progression of IR from adipose tissue-specific pathology [114, 115].

Human genetic research has also suggested that adipose tissue plays a significant role in IR. Studies in identical twins or first-degree relatives of T2D patients have shown that inheritance has a substantial influence in IR and T2D [116]. More than 250 genetic loci have been linked to T2D so far, however they only account for 25% of T2D heritability [117]. While these investigations have generally discovered genes linked to beta-cell function and insulin secretion, deeper analysis of phenotypes more closely aligned with IR have begun to uncover genetic drivers of IR in other organs. Surprisingly, several of these drivers are involved in the function of adipose tissue [118]. Although subclinical lipodystrophy is a rare cause of severe IR, it has been suggested that milder forms of lipodystrophy are responsible for IR in general, supporting a model in which excessive lipid spillover into circulation is a proximal, mechanistic cause of altered insulin action. Specifically, when the individual's capacity to store lipids in adipose tissue has been exceeded, lipid spillover into circulation leads to elevated plasma FFAs and triglyceride levels, which result in increased ectopic storage of these molecules in non-adipose tissues—such as liver and skeletal muscle—and subsequent metabolic derangements via lipotoxicity (lipid-induced toxicity). Surprisingly, genes in the insulin signaling system linked to IR (IRS1 and GRB14) are also linked to familial partial lipodystrophy [119].

PPARG (Peroxisome Proliferator-Activated Receptor Gamma, a master positive regulator of adipogenesis) and CCDC92, DNAH10, and L3MBTL3 (regulators of adipocyte differentiation) were among the 53 loci discovered in a study employing an integrated genomic approach to find genes related to IR. Thiazolidinediones are insulin-sensitizing peroxisome proliferator-activated receptor gamma agonists that are used in the treatment of T2D and act by promoting adipogenesis and adipose tissue growth (through cell size and cell number increase or adipocyte hypertrophy and hyperplasia) [119]. The availability of additional lipid storage induced by thiazolidinediones may therefore promote insulin sensitivity by alleviating lipotoxicity [120]. These drugs also improve insulin sensitivity in first-degree relatives of T2D patients, implying that adipose tissue hypertrophy and "unhealthy" lipid storage are critical regulators of insulin action and contributors to IR [121].

Adipose tissue's primary function is to store fat and release it into circulation when needed, and it has the unique capacity to expand in response to nutrient overload. Lipids can be released into the bloodstream when the adipocyte capacity to store lipids has been exceeded [39]. There is compelling evidence that the accumulation of excess lipids in non-adipose tissues (e.g., skeletal muscle and liver), known as lipotoxicity (a.k.a. lipid-induced toxicity), plays a role in the development of muscle and liver IR [122]. As a result, studies aimed at understanding the cause and magnitude of increased circulating lipid levels in IR are now being pursued. Furthermore, intracellular lipid accumulation in cells and tissues—including pancreatic beta cells and liver—has been linked to the onset of cellular dysfunctions, such as secretory abnormalities and inflammation (**Figure 2**). Elevated circulating FFA levels have been linked to IR, and this has been proposed as a possible cause of lipotoxicity [123].

In humans and animals, lipid infusion causes muscle IR and enhanced hepatic gluconeogenesis, the latter attributable to changes in metabolic fluxes rather than to fat accumulation [123–125]. Furthermore, animals with increased circulating FFA levels due to increased lipolysis develop muscle and hepatic IR, whereas obese mice with reduced fat cell lipolysis are protected from glucose intolerance [126]. It is worth noting that, as discussed elsewhere [127], circulating FFA levels in patients with IR or T2D usually are not elevated. However, there are several confounders in this measurement, including the wide range of FFA levels in healthy adults and the fact that fasting FFAs are typically assessed rather than the more relevant postprandial FFAs. Nonetheless, there is strong evidence that serum FFA levels are elevated in first-degree relatives of patients with T2D [127, 128], implying that this elevation represents an early stage of the disease. It is unclear if the rise in circulating FFA levels is related to defects in insulin-mediated regulation of lipolysis, to alterations in fat

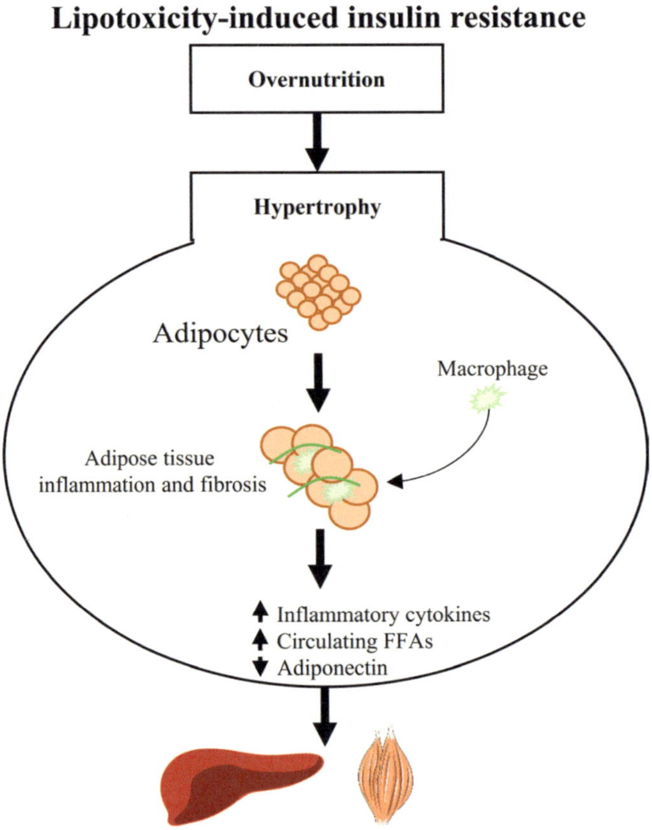

Figure 2.
Excessive adipocyte lipid storage in response to overnutrition, resulting in adipocyte hypertrophy, inflammation and increased release of free fatty acids (FFAs) into circulation, leading to ectopic fat accumulation, lipotoxicity and development of insulin resistance in non-adipose tissues, such as liver and skeletal muscle.

storage capacity, or to an increase in adipose tissue mass without defects in lipolysis. Lipolysis per gram of adipose tissue mass is considerably lower in obese subjects, suggesting that enlargement of adipose tissue mass is the principal driver of abnormal FFA homeostasis [129].

Adipose tissue can grow in size by either hypertrophy, which involves the enlargement of existing adipocytes, or hyperplasia, which involves the generation of new fat cells from preadipocytes via adipogenesis, resulting in an increase in the number of tiny adipocytes [130]. Subcutaneous adipose tissue is more expandable than visceral adipose tissue in humans, whereas the opposite is true in C57BL/6J male mice [131]. Female mice, interestingly, show expandability of both adipose tissue depots in response to Western diet feeding, suggesting that sex hormones and other sex-dependent elements play a role in this process [131, 132]. Pathological adipose tissue expandability under situations of overnutrition, particularly adipose tissue hypertrophy, has got a lot of attention as a likely cause of IR. Indeed, first-degree relatives of patients with T2D have greater amounts of hypertrophic adipose tissue, implying that changes in cell size—presumably due to defective adipogenesis—represent an early event in the pathophysiology of T2D. Hypertrophic large adipocytes are linked to poor metabolic outcomes when compared to hyperplastic adipocytes [39, 133], which have been shown to confer metabolic health in obesity [134–136]. More importantly, hypertrophic adipocytes may contribute to an increase in circulating FFA levels due to their reduced FFA storage capacity. Reduced preadipocyte differentiation, diminished de novo lipogenesis or FFA uptake in hypertrophic adipocytes, and/or reduced adipose tissue expandability due to physical limits on expanding cell size may all contribute to decreased lipid storage capacity by the hypertrophic adipose tissue. Furthermore, adipogenesis abnormalities may result in decreased generation of beige adipocytes, thereby contributing to higher circulating FFA levels; indeed, beige adipocytes differentiate from a subpopulation of progenitors resident in white adipose tissue and have the ability to promote FFA oxidation through thermogenesis [137, 138].

10.2 Circulatory factors released from adipocytes

Adipose tissue secretes a number of factors (termed "adipokines") into the bloodstream that regulate energy metabolism. These factors include cytokines, hormones, extracellular matrix proteins, as well as growth and vasoactive factors. The type of adipose tissue expansion has been demonstrated to impact the secretion of certain of these factors under IR conditions. Since the discovery of leptin as the first adipokine [139], a growing list of adipose tissue-secreted factors implicated in IR has been discovered, with roles in IR that are either protective or causative [20, 140].

Leptin, for example, regulates whole-body energy metabolism by acting on feeding centers in the brain to suppress food intake and increase energy expenditure; leptin deficiency causes obesity, hyperinsulinemia, IR and impaired glucose homeostasis [141]. Adiponectin, another well-known adipokine secreted from adipocytes, has been linked to regulation of cell insulin sensitivity. In humans, circulating adiponectin levels are favorably linked with whole-body insulin sensitivity; additionally, physical training increases circulating adiponectin levels and the expression of its receptors in muscle, which may mediate the improvement of IR in response to exercise [142]. Surprisingly, small and subcutaneous adipocytes release more adiponectin than visceral or large adipocytes [143]. Anti-atherogenic, anti-inflammatory, and insulin-sensitizing effects of adiponectin have also been discovered [144].

It is worth mentioning, however, that while adiponectin's positive benefits in rats are outstanding, the role of this adipokine in humans is less obvious, and Mendelian randomization studies on adiponectin's relationship with metabolic disease in humans have generated inconsistent results [145, 146].

Adipocytes release a variety of substances, including metabolites like lipids and extracellular vesicles that contain proteins and microRNAs. Branched fatty acid esters of hydroxy fatty acids (FAHFAs) are a unique class of lipids synthesized in adipocytes that have been shown to increase insulin sensitivity and reduce inflammation; accordingly, individuals with IR have lower circulating FAHFA levels [147]. As a result, further research into this metabolite class is necessary. Adipocytes, for example, release tiny lipid-encapsulated extracellular vesicles into the bloodstream. These vesicles may alter metabolic processes in other target tissues, such as the liver, according to increasing evidence based on mouse studies. MicroRNAs represent one of the components found in extracellular vesicles that have been linked to this mechanism. While investigations on microRNAs are intriguing, many fundamental aspects about the mechanism of their controlled secretion and their tissue targeting and entry into target cells remain unknown [148, 149].

Many circulating factors are also produced by other adipose tissue-resident cells, such as immune or vascular cells, rather than by adipocytes themselves (the so-called "stromal vascular fraction" of adipose tissue). Some of these adipokines, such as tumor necrosis factor (TNF), resistin or vascular endothelial growth factor (VEGF), are important regulators of tissue homeostasis and may be secreted as a result of adipose tissue enlargement during the development of obesity [150]. Nonetheless, inflammatory cytokines have been widely suggested as possible IR-inducing adipokines, and several of these factors have significant proinflammatory activities [151–153].

11. Inflammation and insulin resistance

It is now well recognized that cells of both innate and adaptive immunity, notably macrophages, infiltrate hypertrophic adipose tissue in most obesity models, and that this is accompanied by a loss of immunosuppressive regulatory T cells in visceral fat depots [154]. When macrophages in adipose tissue are activated in response to overnutrition, they polarize towards a proinflammatory phenotype and release cytokines that may trigger IR in all metabolic tissues [155]. Diet-induced obesity in mice and humans is unmistakably linked to elevated levels of systemic inflammatory markers, including C-reactive protein (CRP) and enhanced immune cell infiltration of adipose tissue and other organs [156]. In addition, inflammatory cytokines, such as TNF, can elicit IR in metabolic tissues when infused in humans [157]. Although macrophage infiltration into hypertrophic adipose tissue is well documented, the role of inflammation in IR is convoluted and controversial; for example, inflammatory markers are not elevated in first-degree relatives of T2D patients [158]. Furthermore, in Western diet-fed mice, tissue IR occurs before the adipose tissue infiltration by a considerable number of immune cells, and genetic or pharmacological anti-inflammatory methods do not prevent the development of Western diet-induced IR [159, 160]. The administration of a neutralizing antibody against interleukin-1 (IL-1), a proinflammatory cytokine implicated in IR, to approximately 4000 patients with T2D and almost 5000 subjects with prediabetes resulted in a significant decrease in CRP levels, as well as in a modest positive effect on cardiovascular outcomes, but without reducing the frequency of new-onset T2D or increasing fasting glucose levels [161–163].

Overall, evidence suggests that adipose tissue infiltration by macrophages is unlikely to be the major cause of IR. Macrophage infiltration into the growing adipose tissue may affect its function in addition to systemic inflammation, but the exact impact of this infiltration is unknown [164]. Anti-inflammatory macrophages (M2), on the other hand, have been shown to promote angiogenesis and preadipocyte differentiation, which aids adipose tissue expansion [165, 166]. The diversity of cytokines, their concentrations, and the timing of their release into the tissue are likely to have a considerable impact on the final biological response, contributing to the observed inconsistent results. The ability of genetically induced adipocyte IR to elicit adipose tissue inflammation adds to the growing body of evidence that inflammation may be a consequence rather than a cause of IR. Hyperinsulinemia has been shown to induce adipose tissue inflammation, implying that the latter is a late event in the IR pathophysiology [30].

12. Intracellular mediators and insulin resistance

Many extrinsic stimuli and genetic alterations can antagonize insulin action in vitro and in vivo, and their investigation has led to the identification of a series of molecules as putative intracellular mediators of IR. In the sections that follow, we will look at the role of a few intracellular components that have got a lot of attention as drivers of IR. It is worth noting that mechanisms of action of these components are not well-established yet, and further research is needed to better understand their role in IR development.

12.1 Accumulation of ceramides

Ceramides have been implicated as IR mediators by a large body of research. Ceramides are essential precursors of most of the complex sphingolipids localized in lipid bilayers, including sphingosine, sphingomyelins, and glucosylceramides. Ceramides accumulate in muscle, liver and adipose tissue of subjects with IR, according to human and animal studies [167–170]. In insulin-resistant tissues, the levels of 16- or 18-carbon chain-length ceramides are raised, whereas the levels of other chain-length ceramides are not consistently changed [171, 172]. Indeed, in adipose tissue from obese subjects, the level of ceramide synthase isoform 6 (CERS6), which synthesizes C16 ceramide, is raised [171]. Surprisingly, the presence of a double bond in the ceramide backbone promotes IR, as ablation of the enzyme responsible for its formation (dihydroceramide desaturase 1) abrogates IR [173]. While it is unclear how specific extrinsic mediators of IR cause increased intracellular ceramide levels, it is possible that excess FFAs serve as a crucial substrates for ceramide biosynthesis [174–176].

Another theory connects intracellular ceramide to levels of circulating adiponectin. Ceramidase activity is found on adiponectin receptors, and lower adiponectin levels in IR may lead to decreased ceramidase activity and, consequently, to higher ceramide levels [177, 178]. AMP-activated protein kinase (AMPK), a major metabolic sensor that regulates mitochondrial biogenesis and metabolism, is activated by adiponectin, potentially regulating ceramide via increased mitochondrial lipid oxidation [179]. By using small-molecule inhibitors or genetic deletion of ceramide-producing enzymes to neutralize ceramide accumulation in metabolic organs, researchers were able to reverse or prevent IR induced by the Western diet in C57BL/6 mice with diet-induced obesity [122]. The relationship between ceramide and decreased insulin action is not univocal, as it is for many possible intracellular mediators of IR. In fact, ceramide suppresses AKT activity, although IR is unlikely to be caused by defects in AKT, which is a proximal arm of insulin signaling (as it has previously been mentioned). Ceramide could be part of a wider, IR-related stress mechanism that leads to mitochondrial dysfunction and to the production of reactive oxygen species (ROS). Ceramide has also been connected to the release of pro-inflammatory cytokines, which have been involved in IR, as it has previously been described [180, 181].

12.2 Accumulation of diacylglycerol (DAG)

Another popular theory for the cause of IR is the accumulation of diacylglycerols (DAGs) in muscle, adipocytes and liver, as a result of elevated serum FFA levels [182, 183]. Protein kinase C (PKC) is recruited to the plasma membrane by DAGs, where it phosphorylates and inhibits insulin receptor kinase activity. While it is quite plausible that DAG levels are elevated in insulin-resistant tissues, a scenario in which DAG-dependent phosphorylation of the insulin receptor is the major cause of IR raises a number of questions. Given the "spareness" of the insulin receptor and proximal signaling intermediates, it is doubtful that IR is caused solely by abnormalities in these components, at least in muscle. In contrast to other insulin-responsive proteins, the stoichiometry of insulin receptor phosphorylation at the region implicated in DAG-mediated IR is low and not detectable by conventional phosphopeptide analysis [79, 104, 184]. PKC deletion in the liver had little effect on whole-body insulin sensitivity in mice, indicating against PKC being a key target of DAG-induced IR in that tissue [79, 104], although this has since been challenged by studies in rats showing that acute knockdown of PKC in the liver protected animals from IR. However, antisense oligonucleotides were delivered systemically, which could target PKC expression in other organs. While technical differences between these studies and others have been suggested as a reason for the discrepancies observed [183], there appears to be enough disagreement about the role of the DAG-PKC-insulin receptor pathway in IR to warrant further investigation and, in particular, validation by multiple independent laboratories [185].

12.3 Mitochondrial dysfunction and reactive oxygen species (ROS)

IR has been linked to a decrease in mitochondrial function. Mitochondrial dysfunction is a term that has been used to describe a variety of mitochondrial phenotypes, including decreased respiratory capacity and ATP production, decreased number of mitochondria, accumulated mitochondrial damage due to defects in mitophagy, and altered mitochondrial morphology caused by changes in mitochondrial fission-fusion dynamics. Many of these alterations are also linked to an increase in mitochondrial ROS generation, which has long been linked to IR [186–188].

It is not unexpected that IR is linked to higher levels of reactive oxygen species (ROS). This is due to the fact that IR is frequently accompanied by a positive energy balance, which leads to an excess of reducing equivalents (NADH and FADH2). This determines a reductive stress on the mitochondrial respiratory electron transport chain, which invariably results in the formation of free electrons and, as a result, in an increased production of various forms of ROS [189]. Furthermore, enhanced ROS production has been found in response to a variety of extracellular stressors linked to IR, including inflammation [190]. Superoxide, H_2O_2, reactive nitrogen andoxidized lipids accumulate in insulin-resistant cells or tissues, and a mitochondria-targeted small molecule transiently produced mitochondrial ROS in muscle and adipocytes, causing IR. As a result, attempts to reduce ROS levels have been proven to reverse or prevent IR in mice [191–194].

Reduced levels of coenzyme Q (CoQ) have recently been linked to IR in humans [44]. In mitochondria, CoQ is a key component of the electron transport chain, transferring electrons from complex I or II to complex III. Furthermore, unlike complex I, CoQ receives electrons directly from the electron-transferring flavoprotein, and this is unrelated to proton pumping or mitochondrial membrane potential, relying only on the availability of oxidized CoQ. Reduced CoQ accumulates, causing reductive stress in complex I, complex II and other dehydrogenases that feed electrons into the CoQ pool, resulting in increased ROS production [195]. As a result, lowering the total CoQ pool [44] will most likely lower the ROS production threshold at a given energy demand-supply ratio. It is also worth noting that FFA oxidation produces far more ROS than carbohydrate oxidation [195]. This is because the electron-transferring flavoprotein feeds a higher proportion of reducing equivalents straight into the CoQ pool during FFA oxidation. Therefore, as lipid metabolism increases, the supply of reducing equivalents outnumbers the demand, lowering the ratio of oxidized to reduced CoQ. This is likely worsened when total CoQ levels are low, as seen in IR [44], resulting in reductive stress and increased ROS production. The mechanism that regulates CoQ levels in IR is unknown. Intriguingly, statins, which are commonly used as cholesterol-lowering drugs, have been linked to IR in humans [196], with the possibility that this relationship is related to the statin-induced reductions in CoQ biosynthesis [44]. Unfortunately, given the low bioavailability of CoQ, oral supplements, which are frequently recommended as an antioxidant strategy, are unlikely to be successful in replenishing the mitochondrial CoQ pool in patients with IR or even in individuals who take statins. Other hazardous intermediates can be generated, in addition to ROS, as a result of mitochondrial respiration abnormalities. Acylcarnitine is an example of incompletely oxidized lipids produced by lipid overload. Acylcarnitine has been reported to accumulate in IR, indicating a deficiency in or an overabundance of the mitochondrial oxidative ability. In this regard, it has been postulated that lipid-induced mitochondrial stress mediates IR, although the exact mechanisms remain elusive [197].

12.4 Insulin resistance associated with stress pathway

Many of the pathways involved in IR pathophysiology, such as those involving ceramides, DAGs or ROS, are now being linked as part of what we call an "intracellular IR stress pathway", according to new evidence. Ceramide, for example, promotes mitochondrial fission and ROS production [198, 199]. In subjects with IR, the quantity of mitochondrial ceramide is higher, and enzymes involved in ceramide biosynthesis have been found in mitochondria [185, 200–203]. Ceramide is involved in apoptosis triggered by mitochondria in some cells, including insulin-producing pancreatic beta cells, but not in other metabolic tissues [204–206]. Ceramide also contributes to endoplasmic reticulum stress, which frequently co-occurs with mitochondrial stress and has been proposed as a driver of IR, where endoplasmic reticulum stress causes JNK activation, which, as previously described, affects the insulin signaling pathway via inhibitory IRS1 Ser/Thr phosphorylation [204–206]. Ceramide also induces PKC, a DAG-regulated kinase, to translocate to mitochondria, activating it and causing mitochondrial damage through an unknown mechanism [207].

Ceramides and DAGs are also biochemically connected; sphingomyelin synthase, for example, converts ceramide to DAG. Finally, in rats, reducing mitochondrial ROS levels with mitochondria-targeted catalase improved insulin sensitivity while lowering muscle DAG levels [208]. The potential connection of many of these suspected IR-causing elements into a dynamic network should help to resolve some of the current debates on this topic.

12.5 Signals from the mitochondria

Despite the interest in mitochondrial dysfunction in IR, it is unclear how intramitochondrial signals, like ceramide or ROS, may cause changes in insulin action, such as impaired GLUT4 translocation, which occurs mostly in the cytosol. The mitochondrial permeability transition pore (mPTP), a multiprotein complex located in the inner mitochondrial membrane, is a promising candidate for "inside-out" mitochondrial signaling because it opens under conditions of mitochondrial stress—most notably involving mitochondrial ROS—to allow molecules to be transported from mitochondria to the cytoplasm [209]. In L6 myotubes, inhibiting mPTP prevented ceramide- or palmitate-induced IR, and mice with defective mPTP opening were protected from diet-induced IR in skeletal muscle [210]. Although at least a part of the impact is attributable to its anti-obesogenic effect, deletion of mPTP in the liver has been shown to protect mice from liver steatosis and IR [211].

13. Conclusions and perspectives

The rising frequency of IR, as well as its crucial involvement in a variety of diseases, demands a greater understanding of the processes behind IR pathogenesis and how they interact with genetics and various surroundings, notably dietary factors. We have attempted to offer an overview of the main mechanisms hypothesized to contribute to IR in this chapter, highlighting both supportive and non-confirmatory evidence when appropriate. Many of the molecules and processes studied as causative in IR, in our opinion, function in series as a connected pathway or a loop rather than acting independently. Unfortunately, there has been a recent trend to describe IR as a dysfunction of insulin signaling, regardless of whether a simultaneous examination of insulin action on glucose metabolism has identified a defect in the latter process. We feel that this method has produced significant problems in the field, and we wish to send a message that simple, unitary errors in proximal insulin signaling are unlikely to be a major cause of IR. Rather, IR develops as a result of a variety of challenges that disrupt cellular homeostasis, resulting in cellular stress that can have a variety of deleterious consequences on insulin signal sensing and transmission.

The difficulty in translating findings from model organisms to humans, particularly in terms of differentiating IR causation from the multiplicity of effects, is a key roadblock in investigating the underpinnings of IR. By discovering causal genetic variants, human genetics holds a lot of promise for tackling this problem. However, genetics can only explain a portion of the pathophysiology of IR. Environmental variables play a crucial role in determining susceptibility to IR development and interact with genetics. Furthermore, the heterogeneity of metabolic diseases like T2D demands detailed phenotyping. Focusing on phenotypes that has better track with IR has proven difficult to achieve in the large cohorts. It is required to identify genetic polymorphisms that only explain a small proportion of disease in the human population. Despite these limitations, a number of genetic loci linked to human IR have been discovered, leading to a renewed focus on adipose tissue enlargement as a critical aspect of IR. However, since IR is a systemic condition, we expect future investigations to discover variations in genes governing multiple cellular processes throughout organs as linked to IR pathophysiology.

A more systematic approach involving large-scale omics to analyze the molecular landscape rather than relying on individual components as causal would be required to gain a better understanding of IR. Moreover, while knockout mice have been critical in characterizing the biochemistry of insulin action, they have also sparked numerous debates. One reason for this is that gene deletions typically result in adaptive processes that are difficult to define and may have limited physiological value, as indicated in a recent study with muscle-specific Akt gene-knockout mice [58]. In animals with both insulin and insulin-like growth factor 1 (IGF-1) receptors removed in muscle, similar adaptation mechanisms have been reported [212].

The ultimate goal of understanding mechanisms behind IR is to develop new, effective anti-IR therapeutic strategies. One key point to consider in this endeavor is whether such therapies would be beneficial if the initial insult—nutritional overload—persists. While IR is typically considered abnormal, as it is linked to a variety of disease outcomes, it is also a prevalent component of many normal physiological states, such as starvation, pregnancy, and hibernation. IR is believed to play a protective or adaptive role in such conditions, supporting survival by saving glucose for the brain and other vital tissues and organs or for the fetus during pregnancy. It is possible that IR has a similar function in metabolic disease. Since the primary metabolic tissues are frequently exposed to potentially harmful quantities of nutrients, IR could be a protective mechanism that helps to prevent tissue nutrition overload [190]. However, this comes at a price, namely concomitant hyperinsulinemia, which is the most serious pathophysiological consequence of IR. Insulin-sensitizing drugs may thus act as a "circuit breaker", reducing hunger, inflammation and IR by suppressing hyperinsulinemia. As a result, we believe there is still a strong need to describe the molecular characteristics that drive IR in order to identify appropriate targets that can break the IR vicious cycle.

Acknowledgements

The authors are also thankful to Guru Nanak Dev University (Amritsar, Punjab, India) for providing various facilities to carry out the present work.

Conflict of interest

The authors declare no conflict of interest.

Author details

Atamjit Singh[1], Nikhita Ghai[1] and Preet Mohinder Singh Bedi[1,2*]

1 Department of Pharmaceutical Sciences, Guru Nanak Dev University, Amritsar, Punjab, India

2 Drug and Pollution Testing Lab, Guru Nanak Dev University, Amritsar, Punjab, India

*Address all correspondence to: preet.pharma@gndu.ac.in

References

[1] Himsworth HP. Diabetes mellitus: Its differentiation into insulin-sensitive and insulin-insensitive types. 1936. International Journal of Epidemiology. 2013;**42**:1594-1598

[2] Jee SH, Kim HJ, Lee J. Obesity, insulin resistance and cancer risk. Yonsei Medical Journal. 2005;**46**(4):449-455

[3] Suzanne M. Insulin resistance and neurodegeneration: Progress towards the development of new therapeutics for Alzheimer's disease. Drugs. 2017;77(1):47-65

[4] Pérez-Tasigchana RF, León-Muñoz LM, Lopez-Garcia E, Gutierrez-Fisac JL, Laclaustra M, Rodríguez-Artalejo F, et al. Metabolic syndrome and insulin resistance are associated with frailty in older adults: A prospective cohort study. Age and Ageing. 2017;**46**(5):807-812

[5] Chawla A, Chawla R, Jaggi S. Microvasular and macrovascular complications in diabetes mellitus: Distinct or continuum? Indian Journal of Endocrinology and Metabolism. 2016;**20**(4):546

[6] Singh B, Saxena A. Surrogate markers of insulin resistance: A review. World Journal of Diabetes. 2010;**1**(2):36

[7] Philipson LH. Harnessing heterogeneity in type 2 diabetes mellitus. Nature Reviews. Endocrinology. 2020;**16**:79-80

[8] Ahlqvist E et al. Novel subgroups of adult-onset diabetes and their association with outcomes: A data-driven cluster analysis of six variables. The Lancet Diabetes and Endocrinology. 2018;**6**:361-369

[9] James DE, Strube M, Mueckler M. Molecular cloning and characterization of an insulin-regulatable glucose transporter. Nature. 1989;**338**:83-87

[10] Birnbaum MJ. Identification of a novel gene encoding an insulin-responsive glucose transporter protein. Cell. 1989;**57**:305-315

[11] Bryant NJ, Govers R, James DE. Regulated transport of the glucose transporter GLUT4. Nature Reviews. Molecular Cell Biology. 2002;**3**:267-277

[12] Tunduguru R, Thurmond DC. Promoting glucose transporter-4 vesicle trafficking along cytoskeletal tracks: PAK-Ing them out. Frontiers in Endocrinology. 2017;**20**:329

[13] Yeh JI, Gulve EA, Rameh L, Birnbaum MJ. The effects of wortmannin on rat skeletal muscle. Dissociation of signaling pathways for insulin- and contraction-activated hexose transport. The Journal of Biological Chemistry. 1995;**270**:2107-2111

[14] Clemmensen C et al. Gut-brain cross-talk in metabolic control. Cell. 2017;**168**:758-774

[15] Rizza RA, Mandarino LJ, Genest J, Baker BA, Gerich JE. Production of insulin resistance by hyperinsulinaemia in man. Diabetologia. 1985;**28**:70-75

[16] Erion KA, Corkey BE. Hyperinsulinemia: A cause of obesity? Current Obesity Reports. 2017;**6**:178-186

[17] Lillioja S et al. Insulin resistance and insulin secretory dysfunction as precursors of non-insulin-dependent diabetes mellitus. Prospective studies of

Pima Indians. The New England Journal of Medicine. 1993;**329**:1988-1992

[18] Vaag A, Henriksen JE, Beck-Nielsen H. Decreased insulin activation of glycogen synthase in skeletal muscles in young nonobese Caucasian first-degree relatives of patients with non-insulindependent diabetes mellitus. The Journal of Clinical Investigation. 1992;**89**:782-788

[19] Hollenbeck C, Reaven GM. Variations in insulin-stimulated glucose uptake in healthy individuals with normal glucose tolerance. The Journal of Clinical Endocrinology and Metabolism. 1987;**64**:1169-1173

[20] Ghaben AL, Scherer PE. Adipogenesis and metabolic health. Nature Reviews. Molecular Cell Biology. 2019;**20**:242-258

[21] Jacob S et al. Association of increased intramyocellular lipid content with insulin resistance in lean nondiabetic offspring of type 2 diabetic subjects. Diabetes. 1999;**48**:1113-1119

[22] Lim K, Haider A, Adams C, Sleigh A, Savage D. Lipodystrophy: A paradigm for understanding the consequences of 'overloading' adipose tissue. Physiological Reviews. 2020;**101**:907-993

[23] Akinci B, Sahinoz M, Oral E. In: Feingold KR, Anawalt B, Boyce A, et al., editors. Lipodystrophy Syndromes: Presentation and Treatment. South Dartmouth (MA): MDText.com, Inc.; 2000

[24] Blüher M. Metabolically healthy obesity. Endocrine Reviews. 2020;**41**:405-420

[25] Thomas DD, Corkey BE, Istfan NW, Apovian CM. Hyperinsulinemia: An early indicator of metabolic dysfunction. Journal of the Endocrine Society. 2019;**3**(9):1727-1747

[26] Pontiroli AE, Alberetto M, Capra F, Pozza G. The glucose clamp technique for the study of patients with hypoglycemia: Insulin resistance as a feature of insulinoma. Journal of Endocrinological Investigation. 1990;**13**:241-245

[27] Marbán SL, Roth J. Transgenic hyperinsulinemia: A mouse model of insulin resistance and glucose intolerance without obesity. In: Shafrir E, editor. Lessons from Animal Diabetes VI: 75th Anniversary of the Insulin Discovery. Boston, MA: Birkhäuser; 1996. pp. 201-224

[28] Gray SL, Donald C, Jetha A, Covey SD, Kieffer TJ. Hyperinsulinemia precedes insulin resistance in mice lacking pancreatic beta-cell leptinsignaling. Endocrinology. 2010;**151**:4178-4186

[29] Alemzadeh R, Slonim AE, Zdanowicz MM, Maturo J. Modification of insulin resistance by diazoxide in obese Zucker rats. Endocrinology. 1993;**133**:705-712

[30] Pedersen DJ et al. A major role of insulin in promoting obesity-associated adipose tissue inflammation. Molecular Metabolism. 2015;**4**:507-518

[31] Templeman NM et al. Reduced circulating insulin enhances insulin sensitivity in old mice and extends lifespan. Cell Reports. 2017;**20**:451-463

[32] Czech MP. Insulin action and resistance in obesity and type 2 diabetes. Nature Medicine. 2017;**23**:804-814

[33] Tan S-X et al. Selective insulin resistance in adipocytes. The Journal of Biological Chemistry. 2015;**290**:11337-11348

[34] Tonks KT et al. Impaired Akt phosphorylation in insulin-resistant human muscle is accompanied by selective and heterogeneous downstream defects. Diabetologia. 2013;**56**:875-885

[35] Brown MS, Goldstein JL. Selective versus total insulin resistance: A pathogenic paradox. Cell Metabolism. 2008;**7**:95-96

[36] Hillgartner FB, Salati LM, Goodridge AG. Physiological and molecular mechanisms involved in nutritional regulation of fatty acid synthesis. Physiological Reviews. 1995;**75**:47-76

[37] Hellerstein MK, Schwarz JM, Neese RA. Regulation of hepatic de novo lipogenesis in humans. Annual Review of Nutrition. 1996;**16**:523-557

[38] Titchenell PM et al. Direct hepatocyte insulin signaling is required for lipogenesis but is dispensable for the suppression of glucose production. Cell Metabolism. 2016;**23**:1154-1166

[39] Hammarstedt A, Gogg S, Hedjazifar S, Nerstedt A, Smith U. Impaired adipogenesis and dysfunctional adipose tissue in human hypertrophic obesity. Physiological Reviews. 2018;**98**:1911-1941

[40] Kolterman OG, Insel J, Saekow M, Olefsky JM. Mechanisms of insulin resistance in human obesity: Evidence for receptor and postreceptor defects. The Journal of Clinical Investigation. 1980;**65**:1272-1284

[41] Anjana RM, Pradeepa R, Unnikrishnan R, Tiwaskar M, Aravind SR, Saboo B, et al. New and unique clusters of type 2 diabetes identified in Indians. The Journal of the Association of Physicians of India. 2021;**69**(2):58-61

[42] Jia Q, Morgan-Bathke ME, Jensen MD. Adipose tissue macrophage burden, systemic inflammation, and insulin resistance. American Journal of Physiology. Endocrinology and Metabolism. 2020;**319**:E254-E264

[43] Turner N et al. Distinct patterns of tissue-specific lipid accumulation during the induction of insulin resistance in mice by high-fat feeding. Diabetologia. 2013;**56**:1638-1648

[44] Fazakerley DJ et al. Mitochondrial CoQ deficiency is a common driver of mitochondrial oxidants and insulin resistance. eLife. 2018;**7**:e32111

[45] Perry RJ et al. Hepatic acetyl CoA links adipose tissue inflammation to hepatic insulin resistance and type 2 diabetes. Cell. 2015;**160**:745-758

[46] Van der Heijden RA, Sheedfar F, Morrison MC, Hommelberg PP, Kor D, Kloosterhuis NJ, et al. High-fat diet induced obesity primes inflammation in adipose tissue prior to liver in C57BL/6j mice. Aging (Albany NY). 2015;**7**(4):256

[47] Ali O. Genetics of type 2 diabetes. World Journal of Diabetes. 2013;**4**(4):114

[48] Minokoshi Y, Kahn CR, Kahn BB. Tissue-specific ablation of the GLUT4 glucose transporter or the insulin receptor challenges assumptions about insulin action and glucose homeostasis. The Journal of Biological Chemistry. 2003;**278**:33609-33612

[49] Kim JK et al. Glucose toxicity and the development of diabetes in mice with muscle-specific inactivation of GLUT4. The Journal of Clinical Investigation. 2001;**108**:153-160

[50] Gancheva S, Jelenik T, Álvarez-Hernández E, Roden M. Interorgan metabolic crosstalk in human

insulin resistance. Physiological Reviews. 2018;**98**:1371-1415

[51] Severinsen MCK, Pedersen BK. Muscle-organ crosstalk: The emerging roles of myokines. Endocrine Reviews. 2020;**41**:594-609

[52] Burchfield JG et al. High dietary fat and sucrose results in an extensive and time-dependent deterioration in health of multiple physiological systems in mice. The Journal of Biological Chemistry. 2018;**293**:5731-5745

[53] Hoehn KL et al. IRS1-independent defects define major nodes of insulin resistance. Cell Metabolism. 2008;**7**:421-433

[54] Copps KD, White MF. Regulation of insulin sensitivity by serine/threonine phosphorylation of insulin receptor substrate proteins IRS1 and IRS2. Diabetologia. 2012;**55**:2565-2582

[55] Kahn CR et al. The syndromes of insulin resistance and acanthosisnigricans. Insulin-receptor disorders in man. The New England Journal of Medicine. 1976;**294**:739-745

[56] Kono T, Barham FW. The relationship between the insulin-binding capacity of fat cells and the cellular response to insulin. Studies with intact and trypsin-treated fat cells. The Journal of Biological Chemistry. 1971;**246**:6210-6216

[57] Kahn CR. Insulin resistance, insulin insensitivity, and insulin unresponsiveness: A necessary distinction. Metabolism. 1978;**27**: 1893-1902

[58] Olefsky JM, Kolterman OG, Scarlett JA. Insulin action and resistance in obesity and noninsulindependent type II diabetes mellitus. The American Journal of Physiology. 1982;**243**:E15-E30

[59] Camps M et al. Evidence for the lack of spare high-affinity insulin receptors in skeletal muscle. The Biochemical Journal. 1992;**285**:993-999

[60] Gumà A et al. Effect of benzyl succinate on insulin receptor function and insulin action in skeletal muscle: Further evidence for a lack of spare high-affinity insulin receptors. Molecular and Cellular Endocrinology. 1993;**91**:29-33

[61] Fehlmann M, Morin O, Kitabgi P, Freychet P. Insulin and glucagon receptors of isolated rat hepatocytes: Comparison between hormone binding and amino acid transport stimulation. Endocrinology. 1981;**109**:253-261

[62] Merry TL et al. Impairment of insulin signalling in peripheral tissue fails to extend murine lifespan. Aging Cell. 2017;**16**:761-772

[63] Czech MP. Cellular basis of insulin insensitivity in large rat adipocytes. The Journal of Clinical Investigation. 1976;**57**:1523-1532

[64] Melvin A, O'Rahilly S, Savage DB. Genetic syndromes of severe insulin resistance. Current Opinion in Genetics & Development. 2018;**50**:60-67

[65] Crouthamel M-C et al. Mechanism and management of AKT inhibitor-induced hyperglycemia. Clinical Cancer Research. 2009;**15**:217-225

[66] Nandi A, Kitamura Y, Kahn CR, Accili D. Mouse models of insulin resistance. Physiological Reviews. 2004;**84**:623-647

[67] Jaiswal N et al. The role of skeletal muscle Akt in the regulation of muscle mass and glucose homeostasis. Molecular Metabolism. 2019;**28**:1-13

[68] Lu M et al. Insulin regulates liver metabolism in vivo in the absence of hepatic Akt and Foxo1. Nature Medicine. 2012;**18**:388-395

[69] Tan S-X et al. Amplification and demultiplexing in insulin-regulated Akt protein kinase pathway in adipocytes. The Journal of Biological Chemistry. 2012;**287**:6128-6138

[70] Ng Y et al. Cluster analysis of insulin action in adipocytes reveals a key role for Akt at the plasma membrane. The Journal of Biological Chemistry. 2010;**285**:2245-2257

[71] Larance M et al. Global phosphoproteomics identifies a major role for AKT and 14-3-3 in regulating EDC3. Molecular & Cellular Proteomics. 2010;**9**:682-694

[72] Trefely S et al. Kinome screen identifies PFKFB3 and glucose metabolism as important regulators of the insulin/insulin-like growth factor (IGF)-1 signaling pathway. The Journal of Biological Chemistry. 2015;**290**:25834-25846

[73] Ricort JM, Tanti JF, Van Obberghen E, Le Marchand-Brustel Y. Alterations in insulin signalling pathway induced by prolonged insulin treatment of 3T3-L1 adipocytes. Diabetologia. 1995;**38**:1148-1156

[74] Kurowski TG et al. Hyperglycemia inhibits insulin activation of Akt/protein kinase B but not phosphatidylinositol 3-kinase in rat skeletal muscle. Diabetes. 1999;**48**:658-663

[75] Oku A et al. Inhibitory effect of hyperglycemia on insulin-induced Akt/protein kinase B activation in skeletal muscle. American Journal of Physiology. Endocrinology and Metabolism. 2001;**280**:E816-E824

[76] Yuasa T et al. Platelet-derived growth factor stimulates glucose transport in skeletal muscles of transgenic mice specifically expressing platelet-derived growth factor receptor in the muscle, but it does not affect blood glucose levels. Diabetes. 2004;**53**:2776-2786

[77] Draznin B. Molecular mechanisms of insulin resistance: Serine phosphorylation of insulin receptor substrate-1 and increased expression of p85alpha: The two sides of a coin. Diabetes. 2006;**55**:2392-2397

[78] Copps KD et al. Irs1 serine 307 promotes insulin sensitivity in mice. Cell Metabolism. 2010;**11**:84-92

[79] Brandon AE et al. Protein kinase C epsilon deletion in adipose tissue, but not in liver, improves glucose tolerance. Cell Metabolism. 2019;**29**:183-191.e7

[80] Deblon N et al. Chronic mTOR inhibition by rapamycin induces muscle insulin resistance despite weight loss in rats. British Journal of Pharmacology. 2012;**165**:2325-2340

[81] Lamming DW et al. Rapamycin-induced insulin resistance is mediated by mTORC2 loss and uncoupled from longevity. Science. 2012;**335**:1638-1643

[82] Friedman JE, Caro JF, Pories WJ, Azevedo JL Jr, Dohm GL. Glucose metabolism in incubated human muscle: Effect of obesity and non-insulin-dependent diabetes mellitus. Metabolism. 1994;**43**:1047-1054

[83] Shulman GI et al. Quantitation of muscle glycogen synthesis in normal subjects and subjects with noninsulin-dependent diabetes by 13C nuclear magnetic resonance spectroscopy. The New England Journal of Medicine. 1990;**322**:223-228

[84] Baron AD, Laakso M, Brechtel G, Edelman SV. Reduced capacity and affinity of skeletal muscle for insulin-mediated glucose uptake in noninsulindependent diabetic subjects. Effects of insulin therapy. The Journal of Clinical Investigation. 1991;**87**:1186-1194

[85] Friedman JE et al. Restoration of insulin responsiveness in skeletal muscle of morbidly obese patients after weight loss. Effect on muscle glucose transport and glucose transporter GLUT4. The Journal of Clinical Investigation. 1992;**89**:701-705

[86] Meyer MM, Levin K, Grimmsmann T, BeckNielsen H, Klein HH. Insulin signalling in skeletal muscle of subjects with or without type II-diabetes and first degree relatives of patients with the disease. Diabetologia. 2002;**45**:813-822

[87] Kim YB, Nikoulina SE, Ciaraldi TP, Henry RR, Kahn BB. Normal insulin-dependent activation of Akt/protein kinase B, with diminished activation of phosphoinositide 3-kinase, in muscle in type 2 diabetes. The Journal of Clinical Investigation. 1999;**104**:733-741

[88] Ramos PA et al. Insulin-stimulated muscle glucose uptake and insulin signaling in lean and obese humans. The Journal of Clinical Endocrinology and Metabolism. 2020;**106**:e1631-e1646

[89] Vind BF et al. Impaired insulin-induced site-specific phosphorylation of TBC1 domain family, member 4 (TBC1D4) in skeletal muscle of type 2 diabetes patients is restored by endurance exercise-training. Diabetologia. 2011;**54**:157-167

[90] Caro JF et al. Insulin receptor kinase in human skeletal muscle from obese subjects with and without noninsulin dependent diabetes. The Journal of Clinical Investigation. 1987;**79**:1330-1337

[91] Garvey WT, Maianu L, Zhu JH, Hancock JA, Golichowski AM. Multiple defects in the adipocyte glucose transport system cause cellular insulin resistance in gestational diabetes. Heterogeneity in the number and a novel abnormality in subcellular localization of GLUT4 glucose transporters. Diabetes. 1993;**42**:1773-1785

[92] Ryder JW et al. Use of a novel impermeable biotinylated photolabeling reagent to assess insulin and hypoxia-stimulated cell surface GLUT4 content in skeletal muscle from type 2 diabetic patients. Diabetes. 2000;**49**:647-654

[93] Garvey WT et al. Evidence for defects in the trafficking and translocation of GLUT4 glucose transporters in skeletal muscle as a cause of human insulin resistance. The Journal of Clinical Investigation. 1998;**101**:2377-2386

[94] Gumà A, Zierath JR, Wallberg-Henriksson H, Klip A. Insulin induces translocation of GLUT-4 glucose transporters in human skeletal muscle. The American Journal of Physiology. 1995;**268**:E613-E622

[95] Dills WL Jr, McDonough GM, Kingsley PB. Glucose-stimulated protein synthesis in rat testis slices: Substrate specificity and effects of insulin and substrate analogs. Biology of Reproduction. 1981;**25**:466-474

[96] Chlouverakis C. The action of glucose on lipolysis. Metabolism. 1967;**16**:469-472

[97] Li J, Houseknecht KL, Stenbit AE, Katz EB, Charron MJ. Reduced glucose uptake precedes insulin signaling defects in adipocytes from heterozygous GLUT4

knockout mice. The FASEB Journal. 2000;**14**:1117-1125

[98] Shepherd PR, Kahn BB. Glucose transporters and insulin action—Implications for insulin resistance and diabetes mellitus. The New England Journal of Medicine. 1999;**341**:248-257

[99] Etgen GJ Jr et al. Exercise training reverses insulin resistance in muscle by enhanced recruitment of GLUT-4 to the cell surface. The American Journal of Physiology. 1997;**272**:E864-E869

[100] Klip A et al. Recruitment of GLUT-4 glucose transporters by insulin in diabetic rat skeletal muscle. Biochemical and Biophysical Research Communications. 1990;**172**:728-736

[101] Kennedy JW et al. Acute exercise induces GLUT4 translocation in skeletal muscle of normal human subjects and subjects with type 2 diabetes. Diabetes. 1999;**48**:1192-1197

[102] Ploug T, van Deurs B, Ai H, Cushman SW, Ralston E. Analysis of GLUT4 distribution in whole skeletal muscle fibers: Identification of distinct storage compartments that are recruited by insulin andmuscle contractions. The Journal of Cell Biology. 1998;**142**:1429-1446

[103] Stöckli J et al. The RabGAP TBC1D1 plays a central role in exercise-regulated glucose metabolism in skeletal muscle. Diabetes. 2015;**64**:1914-1922

[104] Humphrey SJ et al. Dynamic adipocyte phosphoproteome reveals that Akt directly regulates mTORC2. Cell Metabolism. 2013;**17**:1009-1020

[105] Kjøbsted R et al. Intact regulation of the AMPK signaling network in response to exercise and insulin in skeletal muscle of male patients with type 2 diabetes: Illumination of AMPK activation in recovery from exercise. Diabetes. 2016;**65**:1219-1230

[106] Eguez L et al. Full intracellular retention of GLUT4 requires AS160 RabGTPase activating protein. Cell Metabolism. 2005;**2**:263-272

[107] Batista TM et al. A cell-autonomous signature of dysregulated protein phosphorylation underlies muscle insulin resistance in type 2 diabetes. Cell Metabolism. 2020;**32**:844-859.e5

[108] Boden G et al. Excessive caloric intake acutely causes oxidative stress, GLUT4 carbonylation, and insulin resistance in healthy men. Science Translational Medicine. 2015;**7**:304re7

[109] Hauck AK, Huang Y, Hertzel AV, Bernlohr DA. Adipose oxidative stress and protein carbonylation. The Journal of Biological Chemistry. 2019;**294**:1083-1088

[110] Snel M, Jonker JT, Schoones J, Lamb H, de Roos A, Pijl H, et al. Ectopic fat and insulin resistance: Pathophysiology and effect of diet and lifestyle interventions. International Journal of Endocrinology. 2012;**983814**:1-18

[111] Samuel VT, Petersen KF, Shulman GI. Lipid-induced insulin resistance: Unravelling the mechanism. The Lancet. 2010;**375**(9733):2267-2277

[112] Hammarstedt A, Graham TE, Kahn BB. Adipose tissue dysregulation and reduced insulin sensitivity in non-obese individuals with enlarged abdominal adipose cells. Diabetology and Metabolic Syndrome. 2012;**4**:42

[113] Weyer C, Foley JE, Bogardus C, Tataranni PA, Pratley RE. Enlarged subcutaneous abdominal adipocyte

size, but not obesity itself, predicts type II diabetes independent of insulin resistance. Diabetologia. 2000;**43**:1498-1506

[114] Abel ED et al. Adipose-selective targeting of the GLUT4 gene impairs insulin action in muscle and liver. Nature. 2001;**409**:729-733

[115] Vazirani RP et al. Disruption of adipose Rab10-dependent insulin signaling causes hepatic insulin resistance. Diabetes. 2016;**65**:1577-1589

[116] Poulsen P et al. Heritability of insulin secretion, peripheral and hepatic insulin action, and intracellular glucose partitioning in young and old Danish twins. Diabetes. 2005;**54**:275-283

[117] Flannick J et al. Exome sequencing of 20,791 cases of type 2 diabetes and 24,440 controls. Nature. 2019;**570**:71-76

[118] Dimas AS et al. Impact of type 2 diabetes susceptibility variants on quantitative glycemic traits reveals mechanistic heterogeneity. Diabetes. 2014;**63**:2158-2171

[119] Lotta LA et al. Integrative genomic analysis implicates limited peripheral adipose storage capacity in the pathogenesis of human insulin resistance. Nature Genetics. 2017;**49**:17-26

[120] MacKellar J, Cushman SW, Periwal V. Differential effects of thiazolidinediones on adipocyte growth and recruitment in Zucker fatty rats. PLoS One. 2009;**4**(12):e8196

[121] Levin K, Hother-Nielsen O, Henriksen JE, Beck-Nielsen H. Effects of troglitazone in young first-degree relatives of patients with type 2 diabetes. Diabetes Care. 2004;**27**:148-154

[122] Chaurasia B, Summers SA. Ceramides in metabolism: Key lipotoxic players. Annual Review of Physiology. 2021;**83**:303-330

[123] Boden G. Free fatty acids (FFA), a link between obesity and insulin resistance. Frontiers in Bioscience. 1998;**3**:d169-d175

[124] Pereira S et al. Resveratrol prevents insulin resistance caused by short-term elevation of free fatty acids in vivo. Applied Physiology, Nutrition, and Metabolism. 2015;**40**:1129-1136

[125] Felber JP, Vannotti A. Effects of fat infusion on glucose tolerance and insulin plasma levels. Medicina Experimentalis. International Journal of Experimental Medicine. 1964;**10**:153-156

[126] Wang L et al. Adipocyte Gi signaling is essential for maintaining whole-body glucose homeostasis and insulin sensitivity. Nature Communications. 2020;**11**:2995

[127] Karpe F, Dickmann JR, Frayn KN. Fatty acids, obesity, and insulin resistance: Time for a reevaluation. Diabetes. 2011; **60**:2441-2449

[128] Perseghin G, Ghosh S, Gerow K, Shulman GI. Metabolic defects in lean nondiabetic offspring of NIDDM parents: A cross-sectional study. Diabetes. 1997;**46**:1001-1009

[129] McQuaid SE et al. Downregulation of adipose tissue fatty acid trafficking in obesity: A driver for ectopic fat deposition? Diabetes. 2011;**60**:47-55

[130] Jeffery E, Church CD, Holtrup B, Colman L, Rodeheffer MS. Rapid depot-specific activation of adipocyte precursor cells at the onset of obesity. Nature Cell Biology. 2015;**17**:376-385

[131] Jeffery E et al. The adipose tissue microenvironment regulates

depot-specific adipogenesis in obesity. Cell Metabolism. 2016;**24**:142-150

[132] Arner P, Arner E, Hammarstedt A, Smith U. Genetic predisposition for type 2 diabetes, but not for overweight/obesity, is associated with a restricted adipogenesis. PLoS One. 2011;**6**:e18284

[133] Ye J. Regulation of PPARgamma function by TNF-alpha. Biochemical and Biophysical Research Communications. 2008;**374**:405-408

[134] Shao M et al. De novo adipocyte differentiation from Pdgfrβ preadipocytes protects against pathologic visceral adipose expansion in obesity. Nature Communications. 2018;**9**:890

[135] Kim J-Y et al. Obesity-associated improvements in metabolic profile through expansion of adipose tissue. The Journal of Clinical Investigation. 2007;**117**:2621-2637

[136] Shepherd PR et al. Adipose cell hyperplasia and enhanced glucose disposal in transgenic mice overexpressing GLUT4 selectively in adipose tissue. The Journal of Biological Chemistry. 1993;**268**:22243-22246

[137] Carobbio S, Pellegrinelli V, Vidal-Puig A. Adipose tissue function and expandability as determinants of lipotoxicity and the metabolic syndrome. Advances in Experimental Medicine and Biology. 2017;**960**:161-196

[138] Czech MP. Mechanisms of insulin resistance related to white, beige, and brown adipocytes. Molecular Metabolism. 2020;**34**:27-42

[139] Zhang Y et al. Positional cloning of the mouse obese gene and its human homologue. Nature. 1994;**372**:425-432

[140] Kahn CR, Wang G, Lee KY. Altered adipose tissue and adipocyte function in the pathogenesis of metabolic syndrome. The Journal of Clinical Investigation. 2019;**129**:3990-4000

[141] Friedman JM. Leptin and the endocrine control of energy balance. Nature Metabolism. 2019;**1**:754-764

[142] Blüher M et al. Circulating adiponectin and expression of adiponectin receptors in human skeletal muscle: Associations with metabolic parameters and insulin resistance and regulation by physical training. The Journal of Clinical Endocrinology and Metabolism. 2006;**91**:2310-2316

[143] Meyer LK, Ciaraldi TP, Henry RR, Wittgrove AC, Phillips SA. Adipose tissue depot and cell size dependency of adiponectin synthesis and secretion in human obesity. Adipocytes. 2013;**2**:217-226

[144] Yamauchi T et al. Targeted disruption of AdipoR1 and AdipoR2 causes abrogation of adiponectin binding and metabolic actions. Nature Medicine. 2007;**13**:332-339

[145] Chen Z et al. Effects of adiponectin on T2DM and glucose homeostasis: A mendelian randomization study. Diabetes, Metabolic Syndrome and Obesity. 2020;**13**:1771-1784

[146] Ortega Moreno L et al. Evidence of a causal relationship between high serum adiponectin levels and increased cardiovascular mortality rate in patients with type 2 diabetes. Cardiovascular Diabetology. 2016;**15**:17

[147] Yore MM et al. Discovery of a class of endogenous mammalian lipids with anti-diabetic and antiinflammatory effects. Cell. 2014;**159**:318-332

[148] Mori MA, Ludwig RG, Garcia-Martin R, Brandão BB, Kahn CR.

Extracellular miRNAs: From biomarkers to mediators of physiology and disease. Cell Metabolism. 2019;**30**(4):656-673

[149] Agbu P, Carthew RW. MicroRNA-mediated regulation of glucose and lipid metabolism. Nature Reviews. Molecular Cell Biology. 2021;**22**:425-438

[150] Crewe C, An YA, Scherer PE. The ominous triad of adipose tissue dysfunction: Inflammation, fibrosis, and impaired angiogenesis. The Journal of Clinical Investigation. 2017;**127**:74-82

[151] Hotamisligil GS. Inflammation and metabolic disorders. Nature. 2006;**444**:860-867

[152] Kammoun HL, Kraakman MJ, Febbraio MA. Adipose tissue inflammation in glucose metabolism. Reviews in Endocrine & Metabolic Disorders. 2014;**15**:31-44

[153] McNelis JC, Olefsky JM. Macrophages, immunity, and metabolic disease. Immunity. 2014;**41**:36-48

[154] Mathis D. Immunological goings-on in visceral adipose tissue. Cell Metabolism. 2013;**17**:851-859

[155] Hotamisligil GS. Inflammation, metaflammation and immunometabolic disorders. Nature. 2017;**542**:177-185

[156] Wu H, Ballantyne CM. Metabolic inflammation and insulin resistance in obesity. Circulation Research. 2020;**126**:1549-1564

[157] Krogh-Madsen R, Plomgaard P, Møller K, Mittendorfer B, Pedersen BK. Influence of TNF-alpha and IL-6 infusions on insulin sensitivity and expression of IL-18 in humans. American Journal of Physiology. Endocrinology and Metabolism. 2006;**291**:E108-E114

[158] Kriketos AD et al. Inflammation, insulin resistance, and adiposity: A study of first-degree relatives of type 2 diabetic subjects. Diabetes Care. 2004;**27**:2033-2040

[159] Shimobayashi M et al. Insulin resistance causes inflammation in adipose tissue. The Journal of Clinical Investigation. 2018;**128**:1538-1550

[160] Lee YS et al. Inflammation is necessary for long-term but not short-term high-fat diet-induced insulin resistance. Diabetes. 2011;**60**:2474-2483

[161] Rafiq S et al. Gene variants influencing measures of inflammation or predisposing to autoimmune and inflammatory diseases are not associated with the risk of type 2 diabetes. Diabetologia. 2008;**51**:2205-2213

[162] Everett BM et al. Anti-inflammatory therapy with canakinumab for the prevention and management of diabetes. Journal of the American College of Cardiology. 2018;**71**:2392-2401

[163] Ridker PM et al. Antiinflammatory therapy with canakinumab for atherosclerotic disease. The New England Journal of Medicine. 2017;**377**:1119-1131

[164] Smith U, Li Q, Rydén M, Spalding KL. Cellular senescence and its role in white adipose tissue. International Journal of Obesity. 2021;**45**:934-943

[165] WernstedtAsterholm I et al. Adipocyte inflammation is essential for healthy adipose tissue expansion and remodeling. Cell Metabolism. 2014;**20**:103-118

[166] Cox AR, Chernis N, Masschelin PM, Hartig SM. Immune cells gate white adipose tissue expansion. Endocrinology. 2019;**160**:1645-1658

[167] Chaurasia B, Summers SA. Ceramides—lipotoxic inducers of metabolic disorders. Trends in Endocrinology and Metabolism. 2015;**26**:538-550

[168] Luukkonen PK et al. Hepatic ceramides dissociate steatosis and insulin resistance in patients with non-alcoholic fatty liver disease. Journal of Hepatology. 2016;**64**:1167-1175

[169] Kolak M et al. Adipose tissue inflammation and increased ceramide content characterize subjects with high liver fat content independent of obesity. Diabetes. 2007;**56**:1960-1968

[170] Coen PM et al. Reduced skeletal muscle oxidative capacity and elevated ceramide but not diacylglycerol content in severe obesity. Obesity. 2013;**21**:2362-2371

[171] Turpin SM et al. Obesity-induced CerS6-dependent C16:0 ceramide production promotes weight gain and glucose intolerance. Cell Metabolism. 2014;**20**:678-686

[172] Stöckli J et al. Metabolomic analysis of insulin resistance across different mouse strains and diets. The Journal of Biological Chemistry. 2017;**292**:19135-19145

[173] Siddique MM et al. Ablation of dihydroceramide desaturase 1, a therapeutic target for the treatment of metabolic diseases, simultaneously stimulates anabolic and catabolic signaling. Molecular and Cellular Biology. 2013;**33**(11):2353-2369

[174] Raichur S et al. CerS2 haploinsufficiency inhibits β-oxidation and confers susceptibility to diet-induced steatohepatitis and insulin resistance. Cell Metabolism. 2014;**20**:687-695

[175] Chaurasia B et al. Targeting a ceramide double bond improves insulin resistance and hepatic steatosis. Science. 2019;**365**:386-392

[176] Chavez JA et al. A role for ceramide, but not diacylglycerol, in the antagonism of insulin signal transduction by saturated fatty acids. The Journal of Biological Chemistry. 2003;**278**:10297-10303

[177] Villa NY et al. Sphingolipids function as downstream effectors of a fungal PAQR. Molecular Pharmacology. 2009;**75**:866-875

[178] Mente A et al. Causal relationship between adiponectin and metabolic traits: A Mendelian randomization study in a multiethnic population. PLoS One. 2013;**8**:e66808

[179] Nawrocki AR et al. Mice lacking adiponectin show decreased hepatic insulin sensitivity and reduced responsiveness to peroxisome proliferator-activated receptor gamma agonists. The Journal of Biological Chemistry. 2006;**281**:2654-2660

[180] Cazzolli R, Carpenter L, Biden TJ, Schmitz-Peiffer C. A role for protein phosphatase 2A-like activity, but not atypical protein kinase Czeta, in the inhibition of protein kinase B/Akt and glycogen synthesis by palmitate. Diabetes. 2001;**50**:2210-2218

[181] Fox TE et al. Ceramide recruits and activates protein kinase C zeta (PKC zeta) within structured membrane microdomains. The Journal of Biological Chemistry. 2007;**282**:12450-12457

[182] Lyu K et al. A membrane-bound diacylglycerol species induces PKCε-mediated hepatic insulin resistance. Cell Metabolism. 2020;**32**:654-664.e5

[183] Lyu K et al. Short-term overnutrition induces white adipose tissue insulin resistance through sn-1,2-diacylglycerol/PKCε/insulin receptor Thr1160 phosphorylation. JCI Insight. 2021;**6**:e139946

[184] Gassaway BM et al. PKCε contributes to lipid-induced insulin resistance through cross talk with p70S6K and through previously unknown regulators of insulin signaling. Proceedings of the National Academy of Sciences of the United States of America. 2018;**115**:E8996-E9005

[185] Perreault L et al. Intracellular localization of diacylglycerols and sphingolipids influences insulin sensitivity and mitochondrial function in human skeletal muscle. JCI Insight. 2018;**3**:e96805

[186] Gonzalez-Franquesa A, Patti M-E. Insulin resistance and mitochondrial dysfunction. Advances in Experimental Medicine and Biology. 2017;**982**:465-520

[187] Sangwung P, Petersen KF, Shulman GI, Knowles JW. Mitochondrial dysfunction, insulin resistance, and potential genetic implications. Endocrinology. 2020;**161**:bqaa017

[188] Houstis N, Rosen ED, Lander ES. Reactive oxygen species have a causal role in multiple forms of insulin resistance. Nature. 2006;**440**:944-948

[189] Fisher-Wellman KH, Neufer PD. Linking mitochondrial bioenergetics to insulin resistance via redox biology. Trends in Endocrinology and Metabolism. 2012;**23**:142-153

[190] Hoehn KL et al. Insulin resistance is a cellular antioxidant defense mechanism. Proceedings of the National Academy of Sciences of the United States of America. 2009;**106**:17787-17792

[191] Anderson EJ et al. Mitochondrial H2O2 emission and cellular redox state link excess fat intake to insulin resistance in both rodents and humans. The Journal of Clinical Investigation. 2009;**119**:573-581

[192] Ingram KH et al. Skeletal muscle lipid peroxidation and insulin resistance in humans. Journal of Clinical Endocrinology and Metabolism. 2012;**97**:E1182-E1186

[193] Duplain H et al. Stimulation of peroxynitrite catalysis improves insulin sensitivity in high fat diet-fed mice. The Journal of Physiology. 2008;**586**:4011-4016

[194] Fazakerley DJ et al. Mitochondrial oxidative stress causes insulin resistance without disrupting oxidative phosphorylation. The Journal of Biological Chemistry. 2018;**293**:7315-7328

[195] Boveris A, Oshino N, Chance B. The cellular production of hydrogen peroxide. The Biochemical Journal. 1972;**128**:617-630

[196] Rees-Milton KJ et al. Statin use is associated with insulin resistance in participants of the Canadian multicentre osteoporosis study. Journal of the Endocrine Society. 2020;**4**:bvaa057

[197] Koves TR et al. Mitochondrial overload and incomplete fatty acid oxidation contribute to skeletal muscle insulin resistance. Cell Metabolism. 2008;**7**:45-56

[198] Di Paola M, Cocco T, Lorusso M. Ceramide interaction with the respiratory chain of heart mitochondria. Biochemistry. 2000;**39**:6660-6668

[199] Smith ME et al. Mitochondrial fission mediates ceramide-induced metabolic disruption in skeletal

muscle. The Biochemical Journal. 2013;**456**:427-439

[200] Novgorodov SA et al. Novel pathway of ceramide production in mitochondria: Thioesterase and neutral ceramidase produce ceramide from sphingosine and acyl-CoA. The Journal of Biological Chemistry. 2011;**286**:25352-25362

[201] vonHaefen C et al. Ceramide induces mitochondrial activation and apoptosis via a Bax-dependent pathway in human carcinoma cells. Oncogene. 2002;**21**:4009-4019

[202] Ye R, Onodera T, Scherer PE. Lipotoxicity and cell maintenance in obesity and type 2 diabetes. Journal of the Endocrine Society. 2019;**3**:617-631

[203] Turpin SM et al. Examination of 'lipotoxicity' in skeletal muscle of high-fat fed 0. The Journal of Physiology. 2009;**587**:1593-1605

[204] Kim Y-R et al. Hepatic triglyceride accumulation via endoplasmic reticulum stress-induced SREBP-1 activation is regulated by ceramide synthases. Experimental & Molecular Medicine. 2019;**51**:1-16

[205] Boslem E et al. A lipidomic screen of palmitate-treated MIN6 β-cells links sphingolipid metabolites with endoplasmic reticulum (ER) stress and impaired protein trafficking. The Biochemical Journal. 2011;**435**:267-276

[206] Flamment M, Hajduch E, Ferré P, Foufelle F. New insights into ER stress-induced insulin resistance. Trends in Endocrinology and Metabolism. 2012;**23**:381-390

[207] Sumitomo M et al. Protein kinase Cdelta amplifies ceramide formation via mitochondrial signaling in prostate cancer cells. The Journal of Clinical Investigation. 2002;**109**:827-836

[208] Lee H-Y et al. Mitochondrial-targeted catalase protects against high-fat diet-induced muscle insulin resistance by decreasing intramuscular lipid accumulation. Diabetes. 2017;**66**:2072-2081

[209] Riojas-Hernández A et al. Enhanced oxidative stress sensitizes the mitochondrial permeability transition pore to opening in heart from Zucker fa/fa rats with type 2 diabetes. Life Sciences. 2015;**141**:32-43

[210] Taddeo EP et al. Opening of the mitochondrial permeability transition pore links mitochondrial dysfunction to insulin resistance in skeletal muscle. Molecular Metabolism. 2014;**3**:124-134

[211] Cho J et al. Mitochondrial ATP transporter depletion protects mice against liver steatosis and insulin resistance. Nature Communications. 2017;**8**:14477

[212] O'Neill BT et al. Differential role of insulin/IGF-1 receptor signaling in muscle growth and glucose homeostasis. Cell Reports. 2015;**11**:1220-1235

Chapter 4

Mechanisms of Insulin Resistance during Pregnancy

Martina Leoni, Nathalia Padilla, Andrea Fabbri, David Della-Morte, Camillo Ricordi and Marco Infante

Abstract

Pregnancy is physiologically associated with a gradual increase in insulin resistance, which acts as a physiologic adaptive mechanism to ensure the adequate supply of glucose to the rapidly growing fetus. However, an early adaptive increase in beta-cell glucose sensitivity and beta-cell insulin secretion maintains glucose homeostasis during normal pregnancy. Potential mechanisms behind gestational insulin resistance include hormonal, placental, and genetic or epigenetic factors, as well as the increase in visceral adipose tissue, alterations in gut microbiota, and the concurrent presence of overweight or obesity. In some instances, defects in beta-cell adaptive mechanisms occur, resulting in a substantial exacerbation of insulin resistance and in the possible development of gestational diabetes mellitus (GDM). This chapter aims to provide readers with a basic knowledge of the physiologic adaptations and the possible dysregulations of glucose homeostasis and insulin sensitivity during pregnancy. Indeed, this knowledge is critical to properly identifying women at risk for maternal and/or fetal metabolic complications and tailoring the prevention and treatment strategies for this population. We also briefly discuss the potential factors and molecular/cellular mechanisms accounting for gestational insulin resistance and GDM pathophysiology.

Keywords: pregnancy, insulin resistance, insulin sensitivity, insulin secretion, beta-cell adaptation, placenta, placental hormones, obesity, inflammation, gestational diabetes mellitus, GDM

1. Introduction

Pregnancy is a unique metabolic event characterized by a series of biochemical, anatomical, and physiological changes aiming to ensure the adequate nourishment of the fetus and to prepare the maternal body for lactation. The pregnancy of a healthy woman is physiologically associated with resistance to the action of insulin on glucose uptake and consumption by maternal peripheral tissues [1, 2]. Insulin resistance during pregnancy serves as a physiological adaptation aimed to subsidize the adequate supply of carbohydrates to the rapidly growing fetus, which uses glucose as the main energy source [2]. Data from normal pregnancies of nondiabetic overweight or obese women demonstrated that resistance to the action of insulin on lipolysis and fat oxidation develops during late gestation and disappears postpartum [3]. Yet, during pregnancy, there is a coexisting balance between the physiologic insulin resistance and an adaptive increase in beta-cell insulin production.

This chapter aims to provide readers with a basic knowledge of the physiologic adaptations and the possible dysregulations of glucose homeostasis and insulin sensitivity during pregnancy. Indeed, this knowledge is critical for identifying women at risk for maternal and/or fetal metabolic complications. We also provide a brief overview of the potential factors and molecular/cellular mechanisms accounting for gestational insulin resistance and gestational diabetes mellitus (GDM) pathophysiology, although these are still not entirely clear.

2. Placental hormones and insulin resistance during pregnancy

The placenta undoubtedly plays a critical role in the development of gestational insulin resistance, as it is supported by the fact that glucose homeostasis rapidly restores after the placental expulsion at delivery [2]. The placenta secretes a series of pregnancy-specific hormones called "placental hormones" (e.g., human chorionic gonadotropin (hCG), human placental lactogen (hPL), and human placental growth hormone (hPGH) into the maternal circulation. These hormones and other hormones (e.g., prolactin) are believed to represent a major factor in reprogramming maternal physiology to achieve an insulin-resistant state [4]. Particularly in mid and late pregnancy, there is a substantial rise in insulin resistance that may be secondary to the marked increase in the production of such hormones [5, 6].

In normal pregnancy, the short half-life of many of the placental hormones in the maternal circulation and the weakening of their effects within 24–48 hours after delivery (accompanied by the reversal of insulin resistance) support the role of these hormones in the development of gestational insulin resistance [7, 8]. Interestingly, this also explains why mothers with type 1 diabetes mellitus (T1DM) experience a rapid decline in insulin requirements (toward pre-pregnancy levels) 1 or 2 days after delivery [2, 9]. Moreover, the circulating concentrations of other non-pregnancy-specific hormones (e.g., prolactin, progesterone, estradiol, and cortisol) increase significantly during pregnancy. The increasing amounts of progesterone, cortisol, and prolactin may also contribute to the post-binding defect in insulin action observed during pregnancy [6, 10]. However, no single hormone has been found to completely account for gestational insulin resistance [2].

In addition, some placental hormones can also influence other canonical hormonal axes in light of their structural similarity to hormones found in the nonpregnant state [2]. For instance, circulating concentrations of hPGH (which differs from pituitary growth hormone by 13 amino acids) increase six- to eightfold during gestation. Thus, hPGH gradually replaces the function of the pituitary growth hormone (GH) during pregnancy [4, 11]. Unlike GH, hPGH is secreted tonically rather than in a pulsatile fashion [2, 12]. This results in maternal serum levels of hPGH comparable to circulating levels observed in acromegaly (e.g., 10 times higher than GH outside pregnancy). Hence, hPGH may exert the same diabetogenic effects of the pituitary GH, resulting in insulin resistance and hyperinsulinemia, reduced insulin-stimulated glucose uptake and glycogenesis, and impaired insulin-mediated suppression of hepatic glucose production [2, 13]. Accordingly, transgenic mice overexpressing hPGH to levels comparable to those observed in the third trimester of pregnancy exhibit severe peripheral insulin resistance [14]. Concerning the molecular mechanisms behind insulin resistance in skeletal muscle in response to elevated hPGH values, it has been shown that hPGH increases the expression of the p85α subunit of phosphatidylinositol 3-kinase (PI3K) in skeletal muscle [4]. In turn, the increase in the p85α subunit of PI3K acts as a dominant-negative competitor to forming a PI3K heterodimer with the p110 subunit, thus inhibiting the PI3K activity and attenuating the insulin signaling downstream [4, 15]. Conversely, data on the potential role of hPL and hCG in the pathophysiology of gestational insulin resistance are less univocal [4, 10, 16].

3. Other factors linked to insulin resistance during pregnancy

Apart from increased secretion of placental hormones and non-pregnancy-specific hormones, other factors have been linked to the pathophysiology of gestational insulin resistance. In this regard, the potential relationship between the placenta and insulin resistance has been suggested to be mediated via the secretion of different pro-inflammatory cytokines and adipokines and/or via the release of other substances from the placenta into the maternal circulation [2, 4]. Obesity and other pregnancy-related factors (e.g., exosomes secreted from both the placenta and adipose tissue, specific genetic polymorphisms, epigenetic factors, pregnancy-related increase in visceral adiposity, and altered gut microbiota composition) can further explain the changes observed in insulin sensitivity throughout pregnancy [4, 17–19].

3.1 Obesity and gestational insulin resistance

Obesity represents a growing public health problem that is increasingly affecting women of childbearing age and pregnant women. More than half of all pregnant women in the United States are considered obese, with 8% being extremely obese [20]. Obese pregnant women are likely to experience several complications during pregnancy, as they exhibit a higher risk for GDM, hypertension, and preeclampsia [21].

Increases in maternal fat mass (seen in both lean and obese pregnant women) and obesity play a central role in the development of insulin resistance during pregnancy [22]. As a consequence of increased insulin resistance, lipid metabolism is also affected during pregnancy; it is characterized by a two- or threefold increase in triglyceride and cholesterol concentrations in late gestation [2]. The impaired insulin-mediated suppression of lipolysis (secondary to insulin resistance) also leads to a substantial increase in circulating values of free fatty acids (FFAs) [2, 23], which can result in lipotoxicity, inflammation, endothelial dysfunction, reduced trophoblast invasion, and consequently reduced placental metabolism and function, particularly in obese women who are more prone to central fat accumulation (central obesity) [24].

Insulin resistance during pregnancy can be particularly exacerbated in the presence of preexisting or concomitant conditions (including diabetes, obesity, and physical inactivity), thus posing serious clinical implications for pregnancy outcomes and long-term morbidity for the mother and offspring [2]. For instance, obese women exhibit increased insulin resistance and increased insulin response, as well as higher circulating inflammatory cytokine values compared with non-obese women both before and during pregnancy. The aberrant increase in insulin resistance secondary to maternal obesity leads to a parallel increase in the risk of developing metabolic syndrome-like disorders during pregnancy, such as hypertension, coagulation disorders, hyperlipidemia, glucose intolerance, and GDM [25]. Importantly, an exuberant increase in gestational insulin resistance can also lead to a surplus of lipids and glucose, resulting in fetal overnutrition and subsequent increased risk of metabolic disease later in life [13]. In this regard, excess nutrient supply, suboptimal *in utero* metabolic environment, and alterations in placental gene expression, inflammation and metabolism may also induce metabolic dysfunctions in the offspring, thus generating a vicious cycle of transgenerational obesity and diabetes [24, 26].

4. Glucose homeostasis and changes in insulin sensitivity during pregnancy

Fetal growth and development depend on multidirectional interactions between the mother, the placenta, and the fetus (maternal-placental-fetal triad). In the context of glucose homeostasis, proper maternal metabolic adaptations are needed to ensure nutrient stores for the fetus and to meet the maternal nutrient requirements. Adequate glucose regulation is essential for guaranteeing maternal and fetal health during the three pregnancy trimesters. In this regard, pregnancy is characterized by two distinct physiologic phases, namely: i) an early anabolic phase, which takes place during the early gestational period (specifically, during the first and second pregnancy trimesters) when there is an increase in nutrient storage and deposition of lipids in maternal tissues; ii) a late catabolic phase, which occurs during the third trimester and is characterized by a marked reduction in insulin sensitivity (insulin resistance) and by enhanced adipose tissue lipolysis [27]. Insulin resistance changes over time during gestation, increasing substantially in the last half of the pregnancy and becoming severe in women with maternal diabetes [2].

During the anabolic phase, the mother stores nutrients to meet the maternal, fetal, and placental energy demands of the future catabolic phase (late gestation) and lactation [27, 28]. In particular, the early stages of pregnancy are characterized by increased beta-cell insulin secretion, while insulin sensitivity may decrease, increase, or even remain unchanged during this period [4, 29]. Following the mid stages of pregnancy, fetal glucose requirements start to increase, prompting the placenta to produce hormones (such as hPGH, hPL, and prolactin) that increase maternal insulin resistance and hepatic glucose production in the effort to preserve the maternal to fetal glucose gradient [30, 31]. In late gestation, maternal metabolism shifts to a catabolic state. This catabolic state results in augmented insulin resistance, enhanced lipolysis (due to reduced insulin-mediated suppression of lipolysis), increased hepatic glucose production, reduced maternal adipose tissue depots, and increased postprandial FFA levels. Overall, there is a reduction of insulin-mediated peripheral glucose disposal (by 40–60% compared with pre-pregnancy levels), which is aimed to allow a greater glucose transport across the placenta [30].

In late gestation, insulin action is particularly decreased in skeletal muscle. As the number of insulin receptors on the skeletal muscle cell surface remains unchanged during the entire pregnancy, the reduced insulin sensitivity is considered to be due to a post-receptor defect in insulin signaling cascade causing a consequential decreased ability of insulin to promote glucose transporter 4 (GLUT4) translocation from the cytoplasm to the myocyte surface and to mediate the subsequent glucose uptake in muscle cells [23]. In pregnant women with normal glucose tolerance, reversal of insulin resistance postpartum is accompanied by enhanced skeletal muscle insulin signaling due to increased expression of skeletal muscle insulin receptor substrate 1 (IRS-1) and downregulation of the p85α subunit of PI3K [32]. These changes allow for greater p85/p110 binding to IRS-1 and play a major role in the metabolic adaptation to normal human pregnancy and restoration of insulin sensitivity postpartum [32]. The p85 regulatory unit of PI3K is a key effector enzyme for stimulating glucose uptake in insulin-sensitive tissues. PI3K is composed of the p85 regulatory unit and a catalytic subunit called p110, which need to form a p85-p110 heterodimer and bind to IRS-1 for PI3K activation. Under the action of hPGH, the p85 monomer is selectively overexpressed and competes with the active p85-p110 heterodimer in a dominant-negative fashion for binding to IRS-1, thus decreasing the IRS-1-associated PI3K activity [13]. In turn, this reduction in PI3K activity results in the attenuation of the final step of the insulin signaling pathway, namely in the reduction of GLUT4 translocation from the cytoplasm to the plasma membrane [13].

4.1 Placental glucose transport and physiologic beta-cell adaptation to gestational insulin resistance

The rate of glucose transfer across the human placenta is directly proportional to the maternal-fetal glucose gradient up to maternal glucose concentrations that are well above the physiologic range [33]. As the fetus has very little capacity for gluconeogenesis, maternal glucose represents the main energy source for the placenta and the fetus. Maternal glucose is crucial for normal fetal metabolism and growth [34, 35].

However, passive diffusion of glucose across the placenta is insufficient to meet fetal glucose needs. Thus, facilitated diffusion using a variety of glucose transporters is required for this purpose. Glucose transporters (GLUTs) are members of the GLUT gene family of facilitated-diffusion transporters. They are embedded in the microvillous (maternal-facing) and basal (fetal-facing) membranes of the syncytiotrophoblast, which is the main placental barrier layer [36]. While eight members of the GLUT family have been described in human placental tissue, only glucose transporter 1 (GLUT1) protein has been identified in the syncytium. Basal membrane GLUT1 expression is upregulated over pregnancy, increased in diabetic pregnancy, and reduced in chronic hypoxia, while microvillous membrane GLUT1 expression remains unaffected [36]. It has been reported that transporter saturation in the perfused placenta occurs with glucose concentrations above 20 mmol/L (360 mg/dL) [37].

As we previously mentioned, there is a coexisting balance between physiologic insulin resistance and an adaptive increase in beta-cell insulin production during pregnancy. In early pregnancy, the endocrine pancreas anticipates the increase in insulin resistance that occurs late in pregnancy through an early increase in beta-cell insulin secretion. As peripheral tissues become progressively more resistant to insulin during normal pregnancy, maternal euglycemia is maintained through a 200–250% compensatory increase in maternal pancreatic insulin secretion [4].

This adaptive increase in insulin secretion may occur through different mechanisms. Lowering the threshold for glucose-stimulated insulin secretion (increased beta-cell glucose sensitivity) is the primary mechanism of the adaptation of pancreatic islets to the increased demand for insulin under normal blood glucose concentrations during pregnancy [38]. In addition, there is an increase in beta-cell mass that occurs via beta-cell hyperplasia and hypertrophy processes and via upregulation of insulin synthesis and secretion [39–41]. Placental lactogens have also been suggested to play an important role in beta-cell adaptation during pregnancy, as these hormones increase beta-cell insulin secretion and beta-cell proliferation and survival, and lower the threshold for glucose-stimulated insulin secretion [42].

Interestingly, a pregnancy-induced increase in C-peptide concentrations (associated with improved metabolic control during pregnancy) has also been demonstrated in women with long-term T1DM, even in women with undetectable C-peptide concentrations in early pregnancy [43]. This phenomenon may be related to different factors, such as: i) pregnancy-induced growth promoting factors influencing the rejuvenation of the beta cells; ii) suppression of the immune system; and iii) improvement in metabolic control leading to reduced beta-cell glucotoxicity [44, 45].

5. Defective beta-cell adaptation during pregnancy and gestational diabetes mellitus (GDM)

Gestational Diabetes Mellitus (GDM) is defined as glucose intolerance of various degrees with onset or first recognition during pregnancy, which is not clearly preexisting diabetes [46]. GDM is one of the most common pregnancy complications, affecting around 2–10% of pregnancies in the United States [47]. GDM is believed to result from pancreatic beta-cell dysfunction in women with preexisting insulin resistance [48]. In particular, defects in beta-cell adaptive mechanisms (through which pancreatic islets adapt to the increased gestational insulin demand) lead to the development of GDM. Compared with women with normal glucose tolerance, women who develop GDM undergo a similar degree of reduction in insulin sensitivity and insulin-mediated whole-body glucose disposal with advancing pregnancy (about 50% reduction) [4]. However, women with GDM fail to overcome peripheral insulin resistance with a proper compensatory increase in endogenous insulin secretion [22].

The reduction in insulin receptor tyrosine kinase phosphorylation and receptor tyrosine kinase activity is observed in pregnant women with normal glucose tolerance and in women with GDM. Yet, the latter group does not exhibit a significant improvement in insulin resistance postpartum [2, 22]. The altered reversal of insulin resistance postpartum in women with previous GDM is likely due to inflammation-induced impairment of peripheral insulin sensitivity secondary to the action of placental hormones and pro-inflammatory cytokines and adipokines (such as leptin, adiponectin, tumor necrosis factor alpha (TNF-α), interleukin-6, resistin) affecting the post-receptor insulin signaling pathway [2, 4, 5]. Notably, TNF-α (a pro-inflammatory cytokine produced from monocytes, macrophages, T-cells, neutrophils, fibroblasts, adipocytes, but also from the placenta) has been suggested as a crucial driver of insulin resistance in both pregnant women with normal glucose tolerance and women with GDM, which acts by inhibiting the insulin receptor tyrosine kinase activity via serine phosphorylation of IRS-1 [2, 4, 5, 22, 49]. Additionally, alterations in the placental structure may also negatively influence glucose homeostasis during pregnancy. Indeed, it has been shown that the placental abnormalities most consistently associated with maternal diabetes are represented by an increased incidence of villous immaturity, increased measures of angiogenesis, and increased placental weight [50]. Also, comorbidities such as diabetes and obesity may further negatively impact the placental function and the insulin signaling in the placental tissue [51]. Specific alterations in placental function have been described in the placentas of obese women as compared with the placentas of lean women, namely reduced mitochondrial respiration and adenosine triphosphate (ATP) generation in trophoblast [52].

Friedman *et al.* [53] examined rectus abdominis muscle biopsies obtained during cesarean section from pregnant women with normal glucose tolerance, pregnant women with GDM, and nonpregnant women undergoing elective surgery (nonpregnant controls). Authors found that insulin resistance to glucose transport during pregnancy is associated with a reduction in IRS-1 tyrosine phosphorylation, mainly due to decreased expression of IRS-1 protein. Yet, in women with GDM, there was also a decrease in tyrosine phosphorylation of the insulin receptor beta-subunit that contributed to further decreases in glucose transport activity [53]. Accordingly, Chu *et al.* [54] found that PI3K activity in adipose tissue of patients with GDM was significantly decreased to 82.89% compared with the control group and negatively correlated with the HOMA-IR (Homeostatic Model Assessment for Insulin Resistance).

Women with a history of GDM exhibit an increased 35–60% risk of developing type 2 diabetes mellitus (T2DM) over 10–20 years after pregnancy [47]. Moreover, GDM is associated with an increased risk of fetal complications (macrosomia, polyhydramnios, neonatal hypoglycemia, shoulder dystocia, respiratory-distress syndrome, increased perinatal mortality) and maternal complications (hypertension, preeclampsia, increased risk of cesarean delivery) [47, 55]. One of the most common and serious complications of GDM is macrosomia, which arises from maternal hyperglycemia. High maternal glucose levels cross the placenta and cause fetal hyperglycemia, which, in turn, stimulates the release of insulin by the fetal beta-cells and causes hyperinsulinemia, resulting in subsequent macrosomia (as insulin anabolic properties induce an increased growth rate of fetal tissues) [47]. It is worth reminding that insulin is present in the fetal pancreas as early as the 10th gestational week and in fetal plasma from the 12th gestational week [56–58].

Many risk factors for the development of GDM are similar to those for T2DM. These risk factors include overweight and obesity, excessive gestational weight gain, advanced maternal age, multiparity, family history of T2DM or GDM, polycystic ovary syndrome (PCOS), physical inactivity, GDM in the previous pregnancy, certain ethnicities (including Asian ethnicity), a previous macrosomic child, Westernized diet, genetic polymorphisms, and intrauterine environment (low or high birth weight) [48, 59–65].

Screening for GDM should be performed particularly in at-risk women through a 2-hour, 75-g oral glucose tolerance test (OGTT) performed at 24–28 weeks of gestation. According to the International Association of Diabetes and Pregnancy Study Groups (IADPSG) criteria, the diagnosis of GDM is made if at least one value of plasma glucose concentration is equal to or exceeds the thresholds of 92 mg/dL, 180 mg/dL, and 153 mg/dl (for fasting, 1-hour and 2-hour post-glucose load glucose values, respectively) after performing a 75-g OGTT [66]. All patients with any risk factor for GDM should receive healthy lifestyle counseling to address modifiable risk factors, such as excessive weight gain and physical inactivity, to prevent GDM [67].

Management of established GDM involves lifestyle intervention consisting of diet counseling aimed at limiting glycemic excursions and ensuring appropriate weight gain (weight control), coupled with self-monitoring of blood glucose (SMBG) and promotion of safe and insulin-sensitizing physical activity regimens. Indeed, it is well known that physical exercise induces a rapid increase in the rate of glucose uptake in the contracting skeletal muscles. This augmented membrane glucose transport capacity is due to the recruitment of GLUT4 transporters to the sarcolemma [68].

Pharmacotherapy is usually started when lifestyle intervention alone fails to lead to adequate glucose control in women with GDM. Pharmacological treatment of GDM involves the use of oral antidiabetic medications (metformin or glibenclamide) or, more frequently, exogenous insulin therapy [69, 70]. Indeed, insulin therapy is considered the first-line pharmacologic therapy for GDM, as insulin does not cross the placenta to a significant degree. Fasting hyperglycemia is treated with basal (long-acting) insulin analogs, while postprandial hyperglycemia is treated with rapid-acting (prandial) insulin analogs. Prandial and basal insulin can be used separately or in combination, based on the individual glycemic profile [71].

Remarkably, appropriate treatment of GDM has been shown to reduce the risk of both maternal and fetal complications of GDM, such as macrosomia, large for gestational age newborns, shoulder dystocia, cesarean section, preeclampsia, and respiratory distress syndrome [72]. Finally, prevention and adequate management of GDM are critical to stop the vicious cycle that increases the risk of developing metabolic dysfunctions such as obesity and diabetes in the offspring [26, 73, 74].

6. Conclusions

Normal pregnancy is physiologically characterized by a progressive increase in insulin resistance, which acts as a physiological adaptation aimed to ensure the adequate supply of glucose to the rapidly growing fetus. However, an early adaptive increase in beta-cell glucose sensitivity and beta-cell insulin secretion ensures the maintenance of glucose homeostasis in normal pregnancy. Potential mechanisms underlying the gestational insulin resistance include hormonal, placental, and genetic or epigenetic factors, as well as the increase in visceral adipose tissue, alterations in gut microbiota, and the possible concurrent presence of overweight or obesity. In some instances, defects in beta-cell adaptive mechanisms occur, leading to substantial exacerbation of insulin resistance and possible development of GDM. A basic knowledge of the physiologic adaptations and the possible dysregulations of glucose homeostasis and insulin sensitivity during pregnancy is critical for identifying women who are at risk for maternal and/or fetal metabolic complications and for properly tailoring the prevention and treatment strategies for this population.

Author contributions

MI conceived and wrote the manuscript. ML and NP equally contributed to writing the manuscript. AF, DDM, and CR revised different parts of the manuscript. All authors have read and agreed to the published version of the manuscript.

Conflict of interest

The authors declare no conflict of interest.

Author details

Martina Leoni[1 †], Nathalia Padilla[2 †], Andrea Fabbri[1], David Della-Morte[1], Camillo Ricordi[3] and Marco Infante[1,3,4,5,6*]

1 Department of Systems Medicine, University of Rome Tor Vergata, Rome, Italy

2 Network of Immunity in Infection, Malignancy and Autoimmunity (NIIMA), Universal Scientific Education and Research Network (USERN), Managua, Nicaragua

3 Cell Transplant Center, Diabetes Research Institute (DRI), University of Miami Miller School of Medicine, Miami, FL, USA

4 Section of Diabetes and Metabolic Disorders, UniCamillus, Saint Camillus International University of Health Sciences, Rome, Italy

5 Network of Immunity in Infection, Malignancy and Autoimmunity (NIIMA), Universal Scientific Education and Research Network (USERN), Rome, Italy

6 Adjunct Professor of Endocrinology, UniCamillus, Saint Camillus International University of Health Sciences, Rome, Italy

*Address all correspondence to: marco.infante@unicamillus.org; marco.infante@uniroma2.it

† These Authors contributed equally to the present manuscript.

References

[1] Catalano PM, Roman-Drago NM, Amini SB, Sims EA. Longitudinal changes in body composition and energy balance in lean women with normal and abnormal glucose tolerance during pregnancy. American Journal of Obstetrics and Gynecology. 1998;**179**(1):156-165

[2] Kampmann U, Knorr S, Fuglsang J, Ovesen P. Determinants of maternal insulin resistance during pregnancy: An updated overview. Journal Diabetes Research. 2019;**2019**:5320156

[3] Sivan E, Homko CJ, Chen X, Reece EA, Boden G. Effect of insulin on fat metabolism during and after normal pregnancy. Diabetes. 1999;**48**(4):834-838

[4] Barbour LA, McCurdy CE, Hernandez TL, Kirwan JP, Catalano PM, Friedman JE. Cellular mechanisms for insulin resistance in normal pregnancy and gestational diabetes. Diabetes Care. 2007;**30**(Suppl 2):S112-S119

[5] Kirwan JP, Hauguel-De Mouzon S, Lepercq J, Challier JC, Huston-Presley L, Friedman JE, et al. TNF-alpha is a predictor of insulin resistance in human pregnancy. Diabetes. 2002;**51**(7):2207-2213

[6] Landgraf R, Landraf-Leurs MM, Weissmann A, Hörl R, von Werder K, Scriba PC. Prolactin: A diabetogenic hormone. Diabetologia. 1977;**13**(2): 99-104

[7] Fuglsang J, Sandager P, Møller N, Fisker S, Orskov H, Ovesen P. Kinetics and secretion of placental growth hormone around parturition. European Journal of Endocrinology. 2006;**154**(3):449-457

[8] Lønberg U, Damm P, Andersson AM, Main KM, Chellakooty M, Lauenborg J, et al. Increase in maternal placental growth hormone during pregnancy and disappearance during parturition in normal and growth hormone-deficient pregnancies. American Journal of Obstetrics and Gynecology. 2003;**188**(1):247-251

[9] Roeder HA, Moore TR, Ramos GA. Changes in postpartum insulin requirements for patients with well-controlled type 1 diabetes. American Journal of Perinatology. 2016;**33**(7):683-687

[10] Ryan EA, Enns L. Role of gestational hormones in the induction of insulin resistance. The Journal of Clinical Endocrinology and Metabolism. 1988;**67**(2):341-347

[11] Handwerger S, Freemark M. The roles of placental growth hormone and placental lactogen in the regulation of human fetal growth and development. Journal of Pediatric Endocrinology & Metabolism. 2000;**13**(4):343-356

[12] Fuglsang J, Lauszus F, Flyvbjerg A, Ovesen P. Human placental growth hormone, insulin-like growth factor I and -II, and insulin requirements during pregnancy in type 1 diabetes. The Journal of Clinical Endocrinology and Metabolism. 2003;**88**(9):4355-4361

[13] Barbour LA. Metabolic culprits in obese pregnancies and gestational diabetes mellitus: Big babies, big twists, big picture: The 2018 Norbert Freinkel award lecture. Diabetes Care. 2019;**42**(5):718-726

[14] Barbour LA, Shao J, Qiao L, Pulawa LK, Jensen DR, Bartke A, et al. Human placental growth hormone causes severe insulin resistance in transgenic

mice. American Journal of Obstetrics and Gynecology. 2002;**186**(3):512-517

[15] Barbour LA, Mizanoor ahman S, Gurevich I, Leitner JW, Fischer SJ, Roper MD, et al. Increased P85alpha is a potent negative regulator of skeletal muscle insulin signaling and induces in vivo insulin resistance associated with growth hormone excess. The Journal of Biological Chemistry. 2005;**280**(45):37489-37494

[16] Ma Q, Fan J, Wang J, Yang S, Cong Q, Wang R, et al. High levels of chorionic gonadotrophin attenuate insulin sensitivity and promote inflammation in adipocytes. Journal of Molecular Endocrinology. 2015;**54**(2):161-170

[17] Jayabalan N, Nair S, Nuzhat Z, Rice GE, Zuñiga FA, Sobrevia L, et al. Cross talk between adipose tissue and placenta in obese and gestational diabetes mellitus pregnancies. Frontiers in Endocrinology (Lausanne). 2017;**8**:239

[18] Crusell MKW, Hansen TH, Nielsen T, Allin KH, Rühlemann MC, Damm P, et al. Gestational diabetes is associated with change in the gut microbiota composition in third trimester of pregnancy and postpartum. Microbiome. 2018;**6**(1):89

[19] Mao H, Li Q, Gao S. Meta-analysis of the relationship between common type 2 diabetes risk gene variants with gestational diabetes mellitus. PLoS One. 2012;7(9):e45882

[20] Flegal KM, Carroll MD, Kit BK, Ogden CL. Prevalence of obesity and trends in the distribution of body mass index among US adults, 1999-2010. Journal of the American Medical Association. 2012;**307**(5):491-497

[21] Cedergren MI. Maternal morbid obesity and the risk of adverse pregnancy outcome. Obstetrics and Gynecology. 2004;**103**(2):219-224

[22] Catalano PM. Trying to understand gestational diabetes. Diabetic Medicine. 2014;**31**(3):273-281

[23] Catalano PM. Obesity, insulin resistance, and pregnancy outcome. Reproduction. 2010;**140**(3):365-371

[24] Jarvie E, Hauguel-de-Mouzon S, Nelson SM, Sattar N, Catalano PM, Freeman DJ. Lipotoxicity in obese pregnancy and its potential role in adverse pregnancy outcome and obesity in the offspring. Clinical Science (London, England). 2010;**119**(3):123-129

[25] Catalano PM. The impact of gestational diabetes and maternal obesity on the mother and her offspring. Journal of Developmental Origins of Health and Disease. 2010;**1**(4):208-215

[26] Alejandro EU, Mamerto TP, Chung G, Villavieja A, Gaus NL, Morgan E, et al. Gestational diabetes mellitus: A harbinger of the vicious cycle of diabetes. International Journal of Molecular Sciences. 2020;**21**(14)

[27] Zeng Z, Liu F, Li S. Metabolic adaptations in pregnancy: A review. Annals of Nutrition & Metabolism. 2017;**70**(1):59-65

[28] Ernst S, Demirci C, Valle S, Velazquez-Garcia S, Garcia-Ocaña A. Mechanisms in the adaptation of maternal β-cells during pregnancy. Diabetes Managing (Lond). 2011;**1**(2):239-248

[29] Catalano PM, Tyzbir ED, Wolfe RR, Calles J, Roman NM, Amini SB, et al. Carbohydrate metabolism during pregnancy in control subjects and women with gestational diabetes.

The American Journal of Physiology. 1993;**264**(1 Pt 1):E60-E67

[30] Lende M, Rijhsinghani A. Gestational diabetes: Overview with emphasis on medical management. International Journal of Environmental Research and Public Health. 2020;**17**(24)

[31] Catalano PM, Huston L, Amini SB, Kalhan SC. Longitudinal changes in glucose metabolism during pregnancy in obese women with normal glucose tolerance and gestational diabetes mellitus. American Journal of Obstetrics and Gynecology. 1999;**180**(4):903-916

[32] Kirwan JP, Varastehpour A, Jing M, Presley L, Shao J, Friedman JE, et al. Reversal of insulin resistance postpartum is linked to enhanced skeletal muscle insulin signaling. The Journal of Clinical Endocrinology and Metabolism. 2004;**89**(9):4678-4684

[33] Day PE, Cleal JK, Lofthouse EM, Hanson MA, Lewis RM. What factors determine placental glucose transfer kinetics? Placenta. 2013;**34**(10):953-958

[34] Hay WW. Placental-fetal glucose exchange and fetal glucose metabolism. Transactions of the American Clinical and Climatological Association 2006;117:321-339; discussion 39-40.

[35] Griffiths SK, Campbell JP. Placental structure, function and drug transfer. Continuing Education in Anaesthesia Critical Care & Pain. 2015;**15**(2):84-89

[36] Baumann MU, Deborde S, Illsley NP. Placental glucose transfer and fetal growth. Endocrine. 2002;**19**(1):13-22

[37] Carstensen M, Leichweiss HP, Molsen G, Schröder H. Evidence for a specific transport of D-hexoses across the human term placenta in vitro. Archiv für Gynäkologie. 1977;**222**(3):187-196

[38] Sorenson RL, Brelje TC. Adaptation of islets of Langerhans to pregnancy: beta-cell growth, enhanced insulin secretion and the role of lactogenic hormones. Hormone and Metabolic Research. 1997;**29**(6):301-307

[39] Baeyens L, Hindi S, Sorenson RL, German MS. β-Cell adaptation in pregnancy. Diabetes, Obesity & Metabolism. 2016;**18**(Suppl. 1):63-70

[40] Salazar-Petres ER, Sferruzzi-Perri AN. Pregnancy-induced changes in β-cell function: What are the key players? The Journal of Physiology. 2022;**600**(5):1089-1117

[41] Van Assche FA, Aerts L, De Prins F. A morphological study of the endocrine pancreas in human pregnancy. British Journal of Obstetrics and Gynaecology. 1978;**85**(11):818-820

[42] Sorenson RL, Brelje TC. Prolactin receptors are critical to the adaptation of islets to pregnancy. Endocrinology. 2009;**150**(4):1566-1569

[43] Nielsen LR, Rehfeld JF, Pedersen-Bjergaard U, Damm P, Mathiesen ER. Pregnancy-induced rise in serum C-peptide concentrations in women with type 1 diabetes. Diabetes Care. 2009;**32**(6):1052-1057

[44] Ilic S, Jovanovic L, Wollitzer AO. Is the paradoxical first trimester drop in insulin requirement due to an increase in C-peptide concentration in pregnant type I diabetic women? Diabetologia. 2000;**43**(10):1329-1330

[45] Shah SC, Malone JI, Simpson NE. A randomized trial of intensive insulin therapy in newly diagnosed insulin-dependent diabetes mellitus. The New England Journal of Medicine. 1989;**320**(9):550-554

[46] Buchanan TA, Xiang AH. Gestational diabetes mellitus. The Journal of Clinical Investigation. 2005;**115**(3):485-491

[47] Quintanilla Rodriguez BS, Mahdy H. Gestational Diabetes. Treasure Island (FL): StatPearls Publishing; 2022

[48] Plows JF, Stanley JL, Baker PN, Reynolds CM, Vickers MH. The pathophysiology of gestational diabetes mellitus. International Journal of Molecular Sciences. 2018;**19**(11):3342

[49] Infante M, Padilla N, Alejandro R, Caprio M, Della-Morte D, Fabbri A, et al. Diabetes-modifying Antirheumatic drugs: The roles of DMARDs as glucose-lowering agents. Medicina (Kaunas, Lithuania). 2022;**58**(5):571

[50] Huynh J, Dawson D, Roberts D, Bentley-Lewis R. A systematic review of placental pathology in maternal diabetes mellitus. Placenta. 2015;**36**(2):101-114

[51] Colomiere M, Permezel M, Riley C, Desoye G, Lappas M. Defective insulin signaling in placenta from pregnancies complicated by gestational diabetes mellitus. European Journal of Endocrinology. 2009;**160**(4):567-578

[52] Myatt L, Maloyan A. Obesity and placental function. Seminars in Reproductive Medicine. 2016;**34**(1): 42-49

[53] Friedman JE, Ishizuka T, Shao J, Huston L, Highman T, Catalano P. Impaired glucose transport and insulin receptor tyrosine phosphorylation in skeletal muscle from obese women with gestational diabetes. Diabetes. 1999;**48**(9):1807-1814

[54] Chu Y, Liu W, Cui Q, Feng G, Wang Y, Jiang X. Analysis of phosphatidylinositol 3-kinase activation in the adipose tissue of gestational diabetes mellitus patients and insulin resistance. Journal of Huazhong University of Science and Technology. Medical Sciences. 2010;**30**(4):505-508

[55] Robert MF, Neff RK, Hubbell JP, Taeusch HW, Avery ME. Association between maternal diabetes and the respiratory-distress syndrome in the newborn. The New England Journal of Medicine. 1976;**294**(7):357-360

[56] Obenshain SS, Adam PA, King KC, Teramo K, Raivio KO, Räihä N, et al. Human fetal insulin response to sustained maternal hyperglycemia. The New England Journal of Medicine. 1970;**283**(11):566-570

[57] Rastogi GK, Letarte J, Fraser TR. Immunoreactive insulin content of 203 pancreases from foetuses of healthy mothers. Diabetologia. 1970;**6**(4):445-446

[58] Steinke J, Driscoll SG. The extractable insulin content of pancreas from fetuses and infants of diabetic and control mothers. Diabetes. 1965;**14**(9):573-578

[59] Pu J, Zhao B, Wang EJ, Nimbal V, Osmundson S, Kunz L, et al. Racial/ethnic differences in gestational diabetes prevalence and contribution of common risk factors. Paediatric and Perinatal Epidemiology. 2015;**29**(5):436-443

[60] Li X, Liu X, Zuo Y, Gao J, Liu Y, Zheng W. The risk factors of gestational diabetes mellitus in patients with polycystic ovary syndrome: What should we care. Medicine (Baltimore). 2021;**100**(31):e26521

[61] Chasan-Taber L, Schmidt MD, Pekow P, Sternfeld B, Manson JE, Solomon CG, et al. Physical activity and gestational diabetes mellitus among Hispanic women. Journal of Women's Health (2002). 2008;**17**(6):999-1008

[62] Morisset AS, St-Yves A, Veillette J, Weisnagel SJ, Tchernof A, Robitaille J. Prevention of gestational diabetes mellitus: A review of studies on weight management. Diabetes/ Metabolism Research and Reviews. 2010;**26**(1):17-25

[63] Petry CJ. Gestational diabetes: Risk factors and recent advances in its genetics and treatment. The British Journal of Nutrition. 2010;**104**(6):775-787

[64] Teh WT, Teede HJ, Paul E, Harrison CL, Wallace EM, Allan C. Risk factors for gestational diabetes mellitus: Implications for the application of screening guidelines. The Australian & New Zealand Journal of Obstetrics & Gynaecology. 2011;**51**(1):26-30

[65] Reece EA. The fetal and maternal consequences of gestational diabetes mellitus. The Journal of Maternal-Fetal & Neonatal Medicine. 2010;**23**(3):199-203

[66] Metzger BE, Gabbe SG, Persson B, Buchanan TA, Catalano PA, Damm P, et al. International association of diabetes and pregnancy study groups recommendations on the diagnosis and classification of hyperglycemia in pregnancy. Diabetes Care. 2010;**33**(3):676-682

[67] Koivusalo SB, Rönö K, Klemetti MM, Roine RP, Lindström J, Erkkola M, et al. Gestational diabetes mellitus can Be prevented by lifestyle intervention: The Finnish gestational diabetes prevention study (RADIEL): A randomized controlled trial. Diabetes Care. 2016;**39**(1):24-30

[68] Richter EA, Derave W, Wojtaszewski JF. Glucose, exercise and insulin: Emerging concepts. The Journal of Physiology. 2001;**535**(Pt 2):313-322

[69] Bergel R, Hadar E, Toledano Y, Hod M. Pharmacological Management of Gestational Diabetes Mellitus. Current Diabetes Reports. 2016;**16**(11):118

[70] Holt RI, Clarke P, Parry EC, Coleman MA. The effectiveness of glibenclamide in women with gestational diabetes. Diabetes, Obesity & Metabolism. 2008;**10**(10):906-911

[71] Szmuilowicz ED, Josefson JL, Metzger BE. Gestational diabetes mellitus. Endocrinology and Metabolism Clinics of North America. 2019;**48**(3):479-493

[72] Behboudi-Gandevani S, Bidhendi-Yarandi R, Panahi MH, Vaismoradi M. The effect of mild gestational diabetes mellitus treatment on adverse pregnancy outcomes: A systemic review and Meta-analysis. Frontiers in Endocrinology (Lausanne). 2021;**12**:640004

[73] Dabelea D. The predisposition to obesity and diabetes in offspring of diabetic mothers. Diabetes Care. 2007;**30**(Suppl. 2):S169-S174

[74] Damm P. Future risk of diabetes in mother and child after gestational diabetes mellitus. International Journal of Gynaecology and Obstetrics. 2009;**104**(Suppl. 1):S25-S26

Chapter 5

Dietary Activation of AMP-Activated Protein Kinase (AMPK) to Treat Insulin Resistance

Barry Sears and Asish K. Saha

Abstract

Lipodystrophy is a rare condition that generates lipotoxicity resulting in significant insulin resistance. However, lipodystrophy is only one of many chronic conditions associated with insulin resistance. Insulin resistance is defined as the impaired ability of insulin to activate GLUT4-mediated glucose transport into target cells. The molecular reason for the failure of glucose transport is less apparent. Considering the wide range of chronic conditions associated with insulin resistance, a new potential understanding of insulin resistance in terms of an accumulation of metabolic stressors resulting in the inhibition of 5′ adenosine monophosphate-activated protein kinase (AMPK) may be warranted. Since AMPK is under robust dietary control, nutrition, as opposed to pharmacological strategies, may be more appropriate to activate AMPK to treat insulin resistance in lipodystrophy and any condition associated with insulin resistance. The focus of this chapter is to outline an AMPK-centric theory of insulin resistance and the combination of defined dietary strategies likely to be necessary to activate AMPK to reduce insulin resistance.

Keywords: lipodystrophy, lipotoxicity, insulin resistance, AMPK, anti-inflammatory calorie-restricted diets, omega-3 fatty acids, polyphenols

1. Introduction

Although lipodystrophy syndromes are rare and heterogeneous disorders, they are characterized by a partial or complete loss of adipose tissue. This loss of adipose tissue results in lipotoxicity as body fat infiltrates into organs that are not designed to store fat [1]. These organs that are primarily affected are the liver and skeletal muscle. This lipotoxicity ultimately leads to insulin resistance that is strongly associated with many chronic diseases, including diabetes, cardiovascular disease and neurological disorders [2]. Furthermore, the loss of adipose tissue reduces leptin levels, thus inhibiting satiety signaling, resulting in increased appetite. This lack of satiety leads to greater calorie intake, increasing the metabolic stress in the organs already affected by lipotoxicity. This increased calorie intake leads to a vicious metabolic cycle of increasing diet-induced inflammation. This chapter discusses how dietary activation of AMP-activated protein kinase (AMPK) may attenuate insulin resistance and thus reduce the severity of lipodystrophy. The same dietary technology may also be applicable to treating a wide variety of other chronic conditions associated with insulin resistance.

2. Classification of lipodystrophy syndromes

The prevalence of various lipodystrophy syndromes is relatively rare and are comprised of a heterogeneous group of disorders. These various syndromes can be characterized as (congenital or acquired) generalized or partial lipodystrophies [3–5]. Generalized lipodystrophy is characterized by an almost complete loss of subcutaneous adipose tissue. This loss of adipose tissue results in low leptin levels leading to a significantly increased appetite [6]. Patients with partial lipodystrophy may exhibit excess adipose tissue accumulation in other areas of the body. Lipodystrophy syndromes usually manifest with several metabolic abnormalities associated with severe insulin resistance that include diabetes mellitus, hypertriglyceridemia, and hepatic steatosis which can progress to steatohepatitis.

Acquired lipodystrophy is a frequent side effect of HIV and antiretroviral treatments that can affect the adipose tissue by several mechanisms [7]. Another cause of acquired lipodystrophy syndrome results from cancer treatments using irradiation especially preceding bone marrow transplants [8].

Finally, localized lipodystrophy is often caused by repeated trauma in the same area, such as injections of insulin, corticosteroids, monoclonal antibodies, and antibiotics [9].

3. Lipotoxicity

Regardless of the cause of lipodystrophy, the immediate consequence is an increased deposition of fat in tissues that are not designed to store excess fat. These tissues include insulin-sensitive tissues such as the liver and skeletal muscle. This type of fat is classified as ectopic fat. The result of increased ectopic fat is the disruption of the normal metabolism in these tissues. The disturbance of normal metabolism by ectopic fat is known as lipotoxicity (or lipid-induced toxicity). When

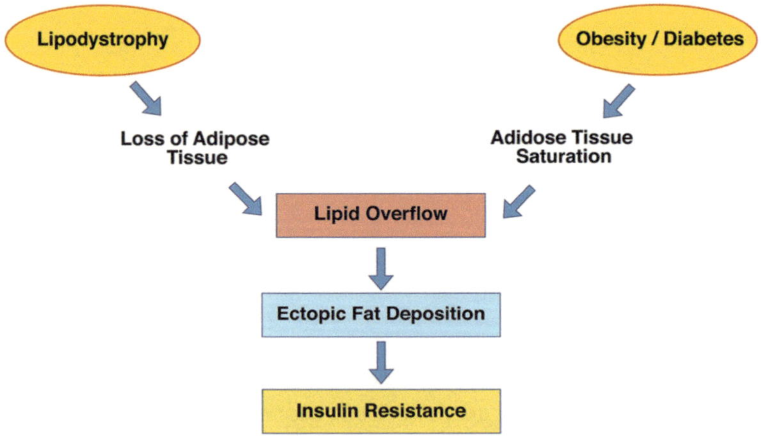

Figure 1.
Lipodystrophy syndromes have been provided critical insights into adipocyte biology and the systemic consequences of impaired adipocyte function. In addition, compelling genetic studies have suggested that subtle partial lipodystrophy is likely a significant factor in prevalent insulin-resistant type 2 diabetes mellitus. In addition, compelling genetic studies have suggested that subtle partial lipodystrophy is likely a significant factor in prevalent insulin-resistant type 2 diabetes mellitus.

lipotoxicity occurs, the ability of these tissues to respond to insulin signaling is compromised, resulting in insulin resistance [10]. Insulin resistance can also occur in other organs such as the brain, where it inhibits insulin signaling in the hypothalamus, that has a crucial role in the regulation of satiety. Insulin resistance in the brain can also reduce the neuronal glucose uptake and use for energy production [11].

Lipotoxicity can also occur when the adipose tissue can no longer expand to store fat safely, leading to fat disposition in the liver and skeletal muscles [12].

Although obesity and type 2 diabetes mellitus are opposite clinical conditions compared to lipodystrophy, they also result in lipotoxicity leading to insulin resistance. In the case of obesity and type 2 diabetes mellitus, adipocytes become saturated with fat and any additional intake of dietary fat or lipids derived from de novo de novo lipogenesis are deposited as ectopic fat in non-adipose tissues. As shown in **Figure 1**, in lipodystrophy, the significant loss of adipose tissue drives any additional dietary fat or de novo synthesized fat to be deposited as ectopic fat in non-adipose tissues. More recently, compelling genetic studies have suggested that subtle partial lipodystrophy is likely to be a major factor in prevalent insulin-resistant type 2 diabetes mellitus [13].

4. Insulin resistance

The concept of insulin resistance was first discussed more than 80 years ago [14]. Insulin resistance can be viewed as the inability of insulin to promote the uptake of glucose into its target tissues. However, its relationship to a larger group of chronic conditions began to be more recognized by the work of Dr. Gerald Reaven [15]. **Figure 2** shows some of the chronic diseases associated with insulin resistance.

Nonetheless, it is still unclear exactly what causes insulin resistance [16, 17]. However, it is known that insulin resistance is also associated with chronic low-level inflammation [18–21].

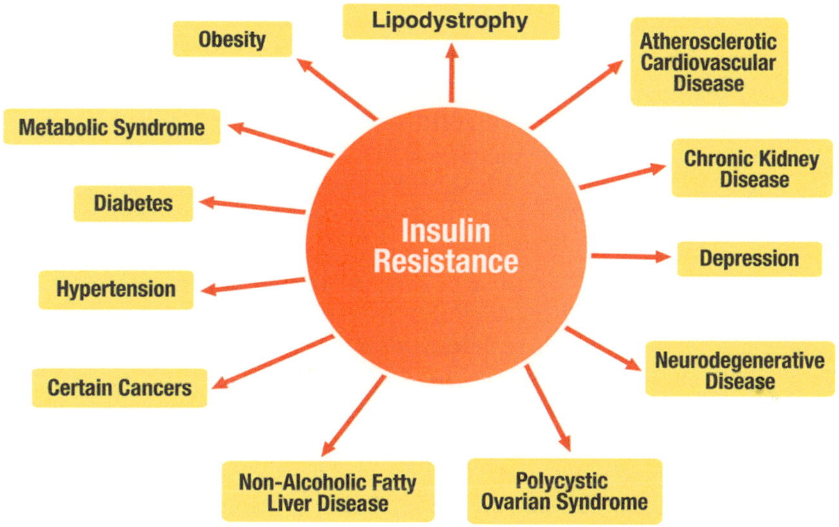

Figure 2.
Chronic diseases that are associated with insulin resistance.

4.1 Putative mechanisms of insulin resistance

The most precise measurement of insulin resistance is represented by the hyperinsulinemic euglycemic glucose clamp [22]. Less precise, but more easily conducted is the use of the HOMA-IR (Homeostatic Model Assessment for Insulin Resistance) test requiring the measurement of both fasting insulin and glucose levels. Other methods of determining insulin resistance would include elevated fasting glucose or elevation in the long-term marker of blood glucose glycated hemoglobin (HbA1c).

On the other hand, determining the intracellular mechanisms that are the underlying cause of insulin resistance has proven more challenging. Randle et al. first postulated that insulin resistance might be caused by fatty acids competing with glucose for substrate oxidation [23]. Through a series of complicated metabolic steps, the result would potentially lead to an increase in circulating glucose levels and decreased glucose uptake by the target cells. Another variation of this mechanism of insulin resistance was the proposed inhibition of glycogen synthase by free fatty acids [24]. In this proposal, insulin resistance occurred primarily in the liver, not in the skeletal muscle.

However, ^{13}C nuclear magnetic resonance spectroscopy experiments seemed to refute this hypothesis, suggesting that much of the glucose uptake occurred in the skeletal muscle [25]. This result shifted thinking on the mechanism of insulin resistance from a glucose-centric theory to a more lipid-centric view. Another potential lipo-centric mechanism has been hypothesized to be the increased production of ceramides in the cell. This proposed mechanism would potentially disrupt the AKT signaling pathway [26]. This would prevent the translocation of the glucose transporter type 4 (GLUT4) to the cell surface needed to transport extracellular glucose into the cell. However, new information on the role of 5′ adenosine monophosphate-activated protein kinase (AMPK) in insulin resistance represented a swing back to a glucose-centric approach [27].

Insulin resistance is also strongly associated with low-level chronic systemic inflammation [28]. One clue of the cause of that inflammation emerged when it was determined that the tumor necrosis factor alpha (TNF-α), a pro-inflammatory cytokine, was associated with insulin resistance [29, 30]. One potential suggested pathway was that TNF-α might inhibit insulin receptor substrate 1 (IRS-1) by phosphorylation [31]. Another proposed variation is that IRS-1 inhibition might be induced by free fatty acids activating the Toll-like receptor 4 (TLR4) on the cell surface [32]. This activation of TLR-4 by free fatty acids would activate NF-κB (nuclear factor kappa B), the master gene transcription factor for inflammation. One of the cytokines produced by an activated NF-κB is TNF-α. This inflammatory hypothesis was reinforced by clinical studies using high-dose aspirin or salsalate to treat type 2 diabetes mellitus [33–35] and c-Jun N-terminal Kinase (JNK) inhibitors to treat insulin resistance [36].

Although there is no current consensus on the molecular cause of insulin resistance, it appears to involve a mixture of lipid, glycemic, and inflammatory stressors in the cells of insulin-sensitive target tissues. The result is making the cell less efficient in taking up glucose from the circulation.

4.2 An alternative mechanism of insulin resistance

As shown in **Figure 2**, many chronic diseases associated with insulin resistance seem to have little direct connection to impairment of the classical insulin signaling system mediated by phosphatidylinositol 3-kinase (PI3K). Therefore, an alternative hypothesis explaining insulin resistance may be via insulin-independent mechanisms that inhibit AMPK activity. AMPK is the master regulator of metabolism in every cell. Therefore, any inhibition of AMPK activity will have significant implications in intracellular metabolism, especially in the reduced ability of the GLUT-4 to translocate to the cell surface and to mediate the glucose transport into the cell for its metabolic needs. It is also known that activation of AMPK increases the phosphorylation of phosphodiesterase 4 (PDE4) [37]. The phosphorylated PDE4 would then inhibit lipolysis in the adipose tissue, thereby decreasing the levels of free fatty acids that would induce greater hepatic glucose production [38]. This would provide another insulin-independent pathway for the reduction of blood glucose levels.

However, controlling the activities of GLUT-4 and PDE4 represents only a limited number of intracellular metabolic processes regulated by AMPK, as shown in **Figure 3**.

These other metabolic actions of AMPK include stimulation of fatty acid oxidation to reduce lipotoxicity and inhibition of NF-κB, which would decrease the production of inflammatory cytokines such as TNF-α. Thus, inhibition of AMPK activity can be related to many of the glycemic, lipid, and inflammatory stressors associated with insulin resistance.

This alternative theory of insulin resistance is reinforced by studies suggesting that the mechanism of PPAR-γ agonists such as the thiazolidinediones (TZDs) - that are used to treat insulin resistance in patients with type 2 diabetes mellitus - may be more due to the activation of AMPK as opposed to the TZDs being ligands of the Peroxisome proliferator-activated receptor gamma (PPAR-γ) [39–42].

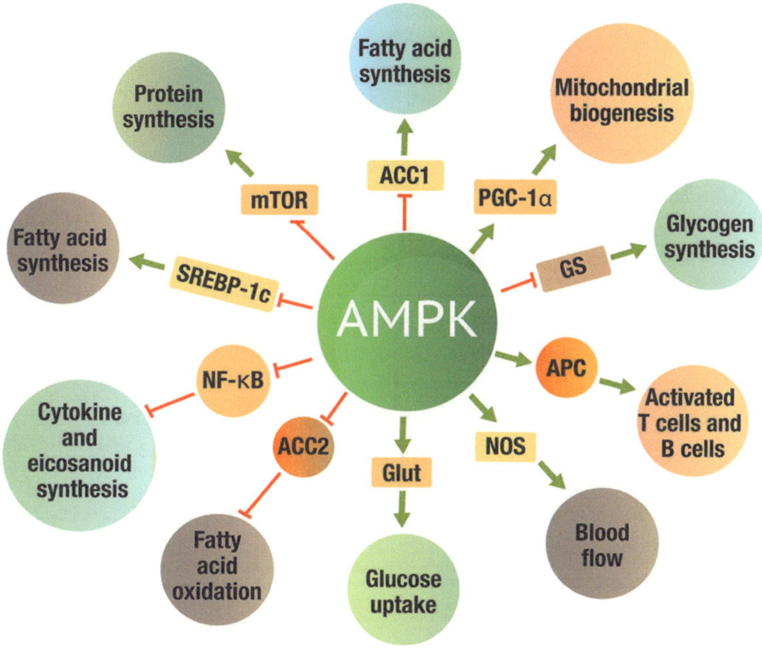

Figure 3.
Metabolic effects of AMPK activation. Green arrows on the "spokes" indicate activation, red lines with a bar at the end indicate inhibition. Abbreviations: ACC1 and ACC2, acetyl-CoA carboxylase 1 and 2; AMPK, 5′ adenosine monophosphate-activated protein kinase (AMPK); APC, antigen presenting cells; Glut4, glucose transporter protein4; GS, glycogen synthase; mTOR, mammalian target of rapamycin; NF-κB, nuclear factor kappa-B; NOS, nitric oxide synthase; PGC-1α, peroxisome proliferator-activated receptor-gamma coactivator 1-alpha; SREBP-1c, sterol regulatory element-binding protein 1c.

It is also known that insulin resistance is strongly associated with reduced AMPK activity [43–46]. Consequently, metabolic disorders such as obesity, metabolic syndrome, type 2 diabetes mellitus, and non-alcoholic fatty liver disease (NAFLD) that are strongly associated with insulin resistance, have been directly linked to decreased AMPK activity [47–49]. Furthermore, other chronic conditions related to increased insulin resistance include hypertension [50], cardiovascular disease [51], polycystic ovary syndrome [52], chronic kidney disease [53], various types of cancer [54], depression [55], and neurodegenerative diseases such as Alzheimer's disease and Parkinson's disease [56]. Each of these conditions can be linked to a decrease in the activity of AMPK.

Since AMPK activity is under robust dietary control, a promising treatment of insulin resistance may be through dietary activation of AMPK [57, 58]. If feasible, such dietary activation of AMPK would increase the transport of GLUT-4 to the cell surface to bring glucose into the cell independent of insulin signaling. In addition, activating AMPK would reduce the levels of accumulated lipotoxic fat by increasing fatty acid beta-oxidation and reducing the production of pro-inflammatory cytokines such as TNF-α via its inhibition of NF-κB activity [59, 60].

Thus, inhibition of AMPK activity could explain many of the clinical manifestations of insulin resistance without invoking the events at the insulin receptor and its downstream signaling pathways as the focal point of the phenomenon of insulin resistance. It would also explain why calorie restriction and exercise are so helpful in reducing insulin resistance because of their direct effects on AMPK activation.

4.3 Drug treatments of insulin resistance

While lipodystrophy is rare, two other metabolic conditions (obesity and type 2 diabetes mellitus) associated with insulin resistance are far more common.

Obesity and type 2 diabetes mellitus initially appear to present a clinical paradox in that they are characterized by excess accumulation of stored fat in the adipose tissue. In contrast, lipodystrophy is a consequence of the loss of adipose tissue [61].

However, all three conditions are characterized by ectopic fat. In the case of lipodystrophy, the accumulation of ectopic fat is caused by a lack of adipose tissue. In contrast, in obesity and type 2 diabetes mellitus, the proliferation of ectopic fat is caused by the inability of the existing adipocytes to store additional fat. Thus, reduction of excess body fat for the treatment of obesity and type 2 diabetes mellitus should be expected with increased AMPK activity. Biopsies of adipose tissue before and after gastric bypass surgery or significant weight loss confirm that the levels of AMPK in the adipose tissue rise significantly [62, 63].

The role of AMPK in reducing insulin resistance in type 2 diabetes mellitus is further suggested because most of the drugs used to treat diabetes operate through activation of the AMPK pathway. These drugs include metformin [64, 65], sodium-glucose cotransporter-2 (SGLT2) inhibitors [66], dipeptidyl peptidase-4 (DPP-4) inhibitors [67] and glucagon-like peptide-1 (GLP-1) receptor agonists [68].

Therefore, a highly structured dietary program that can significantly activate AMPK should be useful in treating insulin resistance, whether it is associated with loss of adipose tissue (i.e., lipodystrophy) or with a reduced capacity of storing excess fat in the adipose tissue (i.e., obesity and type 2 diabetes mellitus).

5. Dietary activation of AMPK

Dietary activation of intracellular signaling pathways is more complex than pharmacology, but it has the advantage of having a far greater therapeutic index. It is more complicated because it usually requires multiple points of dietary intervention to sufficiently activate AMPK and thus greater patient compliance [57, 58]. In essence, there is no single ideal nutrient to optimally activate AMPK to the extent necessary to reduce severe insulin resistance. On the other hand, when using multiple dietary interventions, there is no need to use excessive levels of any single dietary intervention, thereby ensuring an exceptionally high therapeutic index for a dietary program that is likely to be required for a lifetime.

Three specific dietary interventions have the most significant impact on the activation of AMPK: (a) an anti-inflammatory calorie-restricted diet, (b) omega-3 polyunsaturated fatty acids (omega-3 PUFAs), and (c) polyphenols. Although each dietary intervention operates through different mechanisms to enhance AMPK activity, they have significant synergistic interactions [57, 58].

5.1 Anti-inflammatory, calorie-restricted diets

The description of an anti-inflammatory calorie-restricted diet must be highly defined, making it possible to be replicated in controlled clinical studies. This definition includes the total reduction of calories and the macronutrient composition that will increase satiety.

As confirmed by tissue biopsies, calorie restriction remains the most validated approach to activate AMPK [69]. On the other hand, it is usually the most difficult dietary intervention to enhance AMPK activity because it requires dietary compliance. Calorie restriction ideally aims to reduce total calorie intake by 25% of the recommended daily calories needed for current weight maintenance. However, the CALERIE (Comprehensive Assessment of Long-Term Effects of Reducing Intake of Energy) study demonstrated that trying to achieve a 25% reduction by simply reducing calories in young non-obese subjects without adjusting macronutrient ratios of the diet resulted in less than half that calorie restriction guideline being achieved. Nonetheless, significant clinical benefits were observed in the subjects during a 2-year study [70].

Simply restricting total calorie intake ignores the importance of the macronutrient balance of the remaining calories to prevent hormonal disturbances that can lead to increased hunger, loss of lean body mass, and increased inflammation. Protein is the primary macronutrient that needs to be maintained in any type of calorie restriction diet. This macronutrient is essential for improved hunger control and maintenance of muscle mass during calorie restriction. Thus, a calorie-restricted diet should provide about 90 grams of protein per day for an average woman and about 110 grams of protein per day for an average male. Furthermore, this daily protein intake should be evenly spread uniformly throughout the day. This requirement is because the hormonal changes induced by any meal will last only 5 hours before returning to baseline [71]. It has been demonstrated that increased protein intake is also essential to maintain glucagon levels between meals that will help stabilize blood glucose levels, thereby reducing hunger [71]. Another reason is that adequate protein intake is critical for dietary compliance because it enhances the release of gut satiety hormones such as peptide YY (PYY) and GLP-1, further reducing appetite [72]. Thus, consuming adequate protein content at every meal will significantly reduce hunger making long-term calorie restriction more feasible, especially in those individuals with existing insulin resistance [73]. This concept is known as "protein leveraging" [74].

Reducing inflammation requires relatively consistent control of the protein-to-carbohydrate ratio. Regardless of the amount of protein at a meal, it must be balanced by an appropriate level of low-glycemic load carbohydrates to maintain a balance of insulin-to-glucagon in the blood between meals [71, 75]. This balance of insulin to glucagon is also critical in controlling the desaturase enzymes that convert omega-6 fatty acids into arachidonic acid (AA) [76]. Insulin increases the activity of these enzymes, whereas glucagon decreases their activity. Reducing the formation of AA diminishes the potential generation of pro-inflammatory eicosanoids, as AA is the precursor of these eicosanoids. Furthermore, a lower glycemic index of the carbohydrates used at a meal is associated with a lower level of insulin secretion and with reduced AA formation. In addition, low-glycemic index carbohydrates tend to be rich in fermentable fiber that increases the signaling intensity of PYY and GLP-1 from the gut to the appetite control centers in the hypothalamus [77].

Finally, one must consider the total fat content of an anti-inflammatory calorie-restricted diet. First, the fat content should be low because the goal is to activate AMPK to increase the oxidation of existing ectopic fat. Therefore, any excess intake of dietary fat would slow the process. Furthermore, both omega-6 fatty acids and saturated fats can be regarded as pro-inflammatory fats; hence their level should be significantly reduced. The molecular reason is that the omega-6 fatty acids are building blocks necessary for generating eicosanoids, and saturated fats (primarily palmitic acid) can interact with the Toll-like receptor 4 (TLR-4) to activate NF-κB, which will increase the synthesis of cytokines and pro-inflammatory eicosanoids via up-regulation of cyclooxygenase-2 (COX-2) [78]. Therefore, most of the limited fat content of an anti-inflammatory diet should come from monounsaturated fatty acids.

Thus, the definition of an anti-inflammatory calorie-restricted diet becomes decreasing calorie intake by least 500 calories per day below the level estimated to maintain current body weight yet providing adequate protein to maintain lean muscle mass and glucagon levels. That amount of protein is balanced with moderate levels of low-glycemic-load carbohydrates (primarily non-starchy vegetables and limited amounts of fruits). A good starting point for developing the appropriate micronutrient balance of a calorie-restricted anti-inflammatory diet would be about one-third more low-glycemic index carbohydrates to low-fat protein at each meal. Finally, such a diet is low in total fat (especially omega-6 fatty acids and saturated fats) but high in fermentable fiber. Such a diet was first proposed in 1995 [75]. Numerous clinical trials over the years have supported the use of such a defined diet, especially in the treatment of type 2 diabetes mellitus [79–88].

The question is, how long can such a calorie-restricted anti-inflammatory diet be maintained? The answer is potentially indefinitely. The resulting lack of hunger is due to a combination of increased satiety, better control of blood glucose levels to prevent hypoglycemia between meals, and reduced inflammation in the satiety control centers in the hypothalamus. Finally, much of the success in maintaining satiety is based on maintaining a balance of protein-to-glycemic load ratio at each meal [71].

Because a calorie-restricted anti-inflammatory diet is based on protein needs, determining the daily protein requirements for an individual is critical for success. Since the goal is to lose ectopic body fat, but not muscle mass, the subject must consume adequate protein to maintain their existing lean body mass. However, daily protein requirements are not determined by weight, but by lean body mass since total fat mass requires little incoming dietary protein to maintain its biological functions. To determine lean body mass requires determining the total body fat content and then subtracting it from the current body weight. Techniques such bioelectrical impedance analysis (BIA) or dual X-ray absorptiometry (DXA) can accurately determine both compartments [89]. Slightly less accurate measurements can be done by measurement at various body positions. Individuals with a body mass index (BMI) of about 25 Kg/ m^2 have nearly one-third of their total weight as body fat [90]. Since females will have a higher percentage of body fat than males at the equivalent BMI, they have a lower lean body mass and a lower dietary protein requirement to maintain their lean body mass. Although an individual with lipodystrophy will have much lower total body fat levels, the calculation is still the same. Therefore, a good starting point for daily protein requirements for males and females is approximately 1.2 grams of protein per Kg of lean body mass.

Once the protein levels are established based on lean body mass, the levels of carbohydrates and fat needed to fulfill the requirements of the anti-inflammatory component of the calorie-restricted diet are automatically determined. Typically, this diet would be approximately 40 percent of the total carbohydrates coming from low-glycemic index carbohydrates (primarily non-starchy vegetables and limited fruits), 30 percent of the total protein consisting of low-fat protein, and 30 percent of total fat mainly composed of monounsaturated fat sources such as nuts, olive oil, or avocados. This percentage of macronutrients would provide 90 grams of protein, 120 grams of low-glycemic index carbohydrates, and 40 grams of fat for an average female consuming 1200 calories per day or 110 grams of low-fat protein, 150 grams of low-glycemic index carbohydrates, and 50 grams of fat for an average male consuming 1500 calories per day. In addition, since most dietary carbohydrates come from low-glycemic sources, this diet would also be rich in fermentable fiber. Thus, an anti-inflammatory calorie-restricted diet is adequate in protein, moderate in carbohydrates, and low in fat but high in fermentable fiber. Although the levels of carbohydrates are considered moderate in terms of grams, one would need to consume approximately eight servings of non-starchy vegetables and two servings of fruit per day to reach those carbohydrate levels.

However, there are also dietary inhibitors of AMPK. The first of these dietary inhibitors is excess calories. Any calorie-restricted diet makes up for the decreased intake of incoming calories for metabolic needs by the increased oxidation of stored fat. The efficacy of the oxidation of stored fat is ultimately controlled by AMPK activity [91]. Therefore, as one takes in more calories than described above, AMPK activity will decrease, and the oxidation of stored body fat will slow down.

Eventually, there may be a point in time at which excess body fat has been sufficiently reduced. This state is usually indicated by the beginning of the physical appearance of the abdominal muscles that are generally covered by a layer of excess fat. The beginning of the physical appearance of one's abdominal muscles roughly corresponds to a body fat percentage of approximately 22 percent for females and 15 percent for males. These levels of body fat are consistent with being metabolically fit, as stated by the American Council on Exercise. Therefore, if any further body fat loss occurs, one simply adds more non-inflammatory monounsaturated fat to the base calorie-restricted diet until the abdominal muscles are barely perceptible, indicating that the body has an adequate level of stored body fat.

The second dietary inhibitor of AMPK activity would be excess glucose intake. AMPK is also a glucose sensor [92]. Thus, as glucose intake increases, AMPK activity will slow down.

Finally, it has been demonstrated that excess leucine can inhibit AMPK activity in isolated rat skeletal muscle [93]. This inhibition of AMPK by leucine appears to be associated with an increase in lactate/pyruvate ratio and can be overcome by using the pharmacological AMPK agonist 5-aminoimidazole-4-carboxamide-1-β-D-ribofuranoside (AICAR).

5.2 Omega-3 fatty acids

The use of an anti-inflammatory calorie-restricted diet is only one of several specific dietary interventions to enhance AMPK activity. Although helpful in reducing inflammation, the described anti-inflammatory calorie-restricted diet is not very useful for the complete resolution of residual inflammation. The primary dietary component to reach this goal is adequate intake of long-chain omega-3 fatty acids such as eicosapentaenoic acid (EPA) and docosahexaenoic acid (DHA). EPA and DHA are the building blocks for a powerful group of lipid mediators known as specialized pro-resolving mediators (SPMs). These lipid mediators are critical for the resolution of inflammation and stimulating the activity of AMPK by their interaction with specific receptors [94–96]. Therefore, combining adequate omega-3 fatty acids with a calorie-restricted anti-inflammatory diet is synergistic for AMPK activation. A typical starting dosage for omega-3 fatty acids would be 2–3 grams of EPA and DHA per day to make adequate levels of SPMs. For comparison, the average American consumes approximately 100 mg of EPA and DHA per day [57]. Therefore, it is likely that supplementation of omega-3 fatty acids would be needed to activate AMPK.

5.3 Polyphenols

Polyphenols are a class of compounds found in many plant foods that includes flavonoids, phenolic acids, lignans, and stilbenes. Regularly consuming polyphenols is thought to boost digestion and brain health, as well as protect against heart disease, type 2 diabetes mellitus, and even certain cancers [97].

Polyphenols provide a distinct third dietary pathway to activate AMPK [98]. Whereas calorie restriction activates AMPK by energy restriction and omega-3 fatty acids activate AMPK by producing SPMs, polyphenols indirectly activate AMPK by interacting with various sirtuin (SIRT) enzymes. SIRTs are deacetylating enzymes that are activated by polyphenols. Once activated by polyphenols, SIRT1 can facilitate

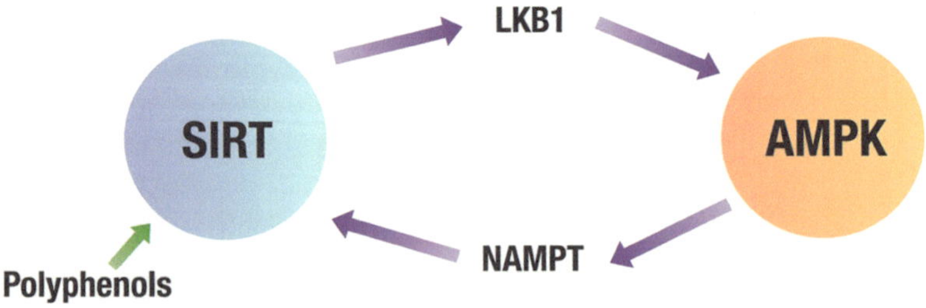

Figure 4.
Crosstalk between SIRT and AMPK. Any decrease in the cell's energy state measured by an increased AMP/ATP ratio will activate AMPK. This activation of AMPK increases NAMPT activity that produces NAD⁺ required for SIRT deacetylation activity. SIRT then deacetylates LKB1, which activates AMPK. Abbreviations: AMP, 5′-adenosine monophosphate; AMPK, 5′ adenosine monophosphate-activated protein kinase; ATP, adenosine-5′-triphosphate; LKB1, liver kinase B1; NAMPT, nicotinamide phosphoribosyltransferase; SIRT, Sirtuins.

the deacetylation of an upstream kinase, liver kinase B1 (LKBT1), promoting the activation of AMPK that increases fatty acid oxidation [99]. An additional benefit is that once AMPK is activated, it will also increase the synthesis of the enzyme nicotinamide phosphoribosyltransferase (NAMPT) to accelerate the salvage pathway to replenish nicotinamide adenine dinucleotide (NAD^+), which is required for continued deacetylation mediated by the SIRT enzymes [100]. This cycle is shown in **Figure 4**.

By increasing NAD^+ levels, the SIRT enzymes can maintain the deacetylation of the p65 Lys310 protein that maintains NF-κB in an inactive state in the cytoplasm, preventing its entry into the nucleus and reducing the synthesis of cytokines and COX-2 enzymes as inflammatory mediators [101].

Another benefit of polyphenol-induced AMPK activation is the increase in the activity of the gene transcription factor nuclear factor erythroid 2-related factor 2 (Nrf2) that will increase the synthesis of various antioxidant enzymes such glutathione reductase and superoxide dismutase [102]. The increase in these antioxidant enzymes will reduce oxidative stress within the cell.

The primary source of dietary polyphenols are fruits and vegetables. Unfortunately, most polyphenols in these food sources are usually either water-insoluble or have polymeric structures. In either case, they will have low bioavailability. However, such polyphenols may be further metabolized into less complex phenolic compounds by the microbiome in the gut. These less structurally complex phenolic compounds may have greater bioavailability but less potential for stimulating the SIRT enzymes. However, some polyphenols (such as monomeric anthocyanins) are directly absorbed and have a more significant impact on activating the SIRT enzymes [103]. If one is supplementing with a water-soluble extract rich in monomeric anthocyanins, a good starting dose would be 450 mg per day. Significant reductions in oxidative stress and oxidation of low-density lipoproteins (LDLs) are observed at this dose [104].

Thus, there are three separate dietary pathways for AMPK activation, as shown in **Figure 5**.

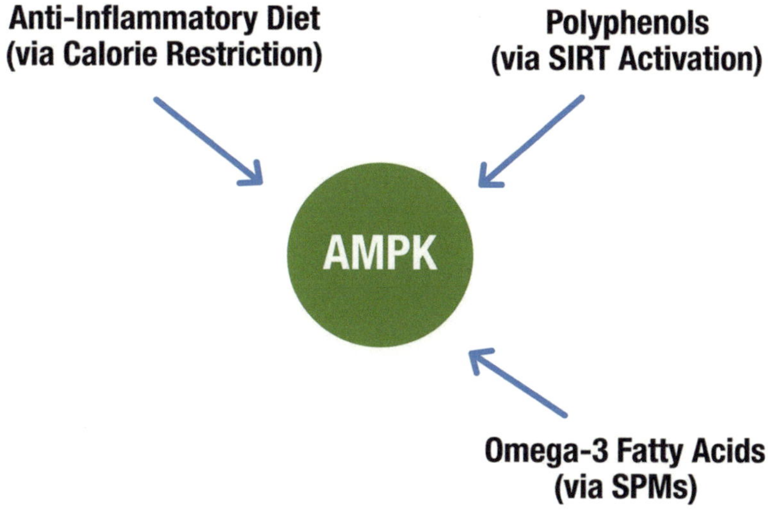

Figure 5.
A graphical description of the dietary interventions that can activate AMPK to reduce insulin resistance. Abbreviations: AMPK, 5′ adenosine monophosphate-activated protein kinase; SIRT, Sirtuins; SPMs, specialized pro-resolving mediators.

Any one of the three dietary pathways is beneficial, but when all three are being used simultaneously, the diet provides a robust but non-toxic methodology to overcome AMPK inhibition. Of these three dietary pathways to activate AMPK, calorie restriction requires the most dietary discipline, whereas adequate intake of omega-3 fatty acids and polyphenols can be easily achieved by supplementation. However, the potential benefits of omega-3 fatty acid and polyphenol supplementation will be significantly attenuated without adequate calorie restriction since excess calories and glucose are dietary inhibitors of AMPK activity. Thus, calorie and glucose restriction become key to ensuring that all three dietary interventions can activate AMPK by working synergistically. Furthermore, using such a synergistic dietary strategy does not require the potential excess intake of omega-3 fatty acids or water-soluble polyphenols to overcome the inhibitory actions of increased calorie or glucose intake that would inhibit AMPK activity.

6. Clinical markers of AMPK activation

Treating insulin resistance using dietary inventions to activate AMPK can be achieved by reducing the intracellular stress on lipid, glycemic, and inflammatory, metabolic responses within the cell. Therefore, the more these three metabolic responses are maintained within appropriate ranges, the greater the degree to which the AMPK becomes activated.

Since AMPK is constrained to remain in the cell, measuring AMPK activity directly without a tissue biopsy is impossible. However, since AMPK is the master regulator of metabolism, several surrogate blood markers can be used to determine whether the dietary interventions described above are achieving their goals of increased intracellular AMPK activity. Such blood markers must be easy to obtain and readily interpreted to make any necessary dietary adjustments to fine-tune them to the individual. The three clinical markers that meet these criteria are the following:

- **Reducing lipid stress**: a primary factor in causing insulin resistance is lipid stress. The triglyceride to high-density lipoprotein cholesterol (TG/HDL-C) ratio is one marker of insulin resistance, especially hepatic insulin resistance [105–112]. Ideally, the TG/HDL-C ratio (measured in mg/dL) should be less than 1.

- *Reducing inflammatory stress*: inflammatory stress is caused by an imbalance in the production of eicosanoids and SPMs. Thus, to maintain an optimal balance of eicosanoids and SPMs, the AA/EPA ratio should be between 1.5 and 3. Within this target AA/EPA range, a significant reduction of various cytokines can be observed relatively quickly [113–115]. Unfortunately, Americans' average AA/EPA ratio is greater than 20 [116, 117], indicating an unfavorable balance of eicosanoids to SPMs. This imbalance fuels the inflammatory component of insulin resistance.

- *Reducing glucotoxicity*: the HbA1c level can be used as a long-term marker of glucose control and glucotoxicity. The HbA1c levels should be maintained between 4.9% and 5.1%, indicating the lack of glucose inhibition of AMPK activity [118].

Only when all three of these three clinical markers are in their proper ranges can AMPK activity be considered optimized for an individual.

It should be noted that optimized AMPK activity differs from continuous AMPK activity. Metabolism is highly dynamic, allowing the cell to adapt to changing conditions rapidly. This optimization using the above-described blood markers enables AMPK to respond to rapidly changing cellular needs for more efficient metabolic activity. In other words, optimization of AMPK activity provides metabolic resilience. If AMPK is constantly active, it can become desensitized to changes in cellular energy status [119]. Maintaining the surrogate blood markers of AMPK activity within these operating limits allows AMPK to retain the necessary metabolic resilience required for maintaining cellular homeostasis.

Specific dietary interventions can modulate each surrogate blood marker of intracellular AMPK activity. For example, the TG/HDL-C ratio can be significantly reduced by following a calorie-restricted diet for 6 weeks [120]. In addition, the dietary intake of omega-3 fatty acids strongly influences the AA/EPA ratio in relatively short periods of time [113, 114]. Finally, the dietary intake of polyphenols to activate AMPK will significantly reduce HbA1c levels within 3 months in pre-diabetic subjects [121]. Furthermore, there is significant crosstalk of the various dietary components as they become synergistic in their cumulative actions [58].

7. Clinical examples of dietary modulation of AMPK activity

Numerous clinical examples demonstrate that the individual dietary interventions described above are effective in chronic conditions characterized by insulin resistance.

7.1 Anti-inflammatory calorie-restricted diets

Numerous examples of treating type 2 diabetes mellitus with an anti-inflammatory calorie-restricted diet have been described [80, 83, 85–88]. In addition, some of the studies range up to 5 years in duration, indicating long-term compliance using an anti-inflammatory calorie-restricted diet is possible [84].

7.2 Omega-3 fatty acids

High-dose omega-3 fatty acids have successfully treated NAFLD, which is a common complication of severe insulin resistance [122]. It has also been demonstrated that an adequate intake of omega-3 fatty acids can cause a statistically significant reduction in pro-inflammatory cytokines [113, 114]. The decrease in pro-inflammatory cytokine levels is likely the result of increased AMPK activity that would inhibit NF-κB activity.

7.3 Polyphenols

Supplementation with monomeric delphinidins (one class of anthocyanins) has been shown to reduce HbA1c in pre-diabetic individuals [121]. This clinical result suggests an increase in AMPK activity that would be consistent with the increase in GLUT-4 transport to the cell surface. In addition, higher doses of monomeric delphinidins also reduce oxidative stress in smokers [104]. This decrease in oxidative stress is most likely mediated by increased AMPK activity that would increase Nrf2-mediated up-regulation of antioxidant enzymes [102].

These clinical examples used only a single dietary intervention to activate AMPK. Thus, it might be reasonably expected that combinations of any two or ideally all three dietary interventions described above would have synergistic effects on reducing insulin resistance.

8. Treating insulin resistance using systems-based biology

Systems-based biology is based on the interconnected signaling pathways within the cell that are required to maintain homeostasis. Furthermore, homeostasis requires rapidly switching from anabolic to catabolic states for cell maintenance. Because of these complex intracellular signaling relationships, a pharmaceutical intervention focused on one pathway may adversely affect other intracellular signaling pathways in the same cell, thereby generating significant side effects.

Our working hypothesis is that dietary activation of AMPK can effectively coordinate these intracellular pathways to decrease various metabolic stresses within the cell that drive insulin resistance. How AMPK activity is intimately connected to many of these diverse signaling pathways is shown in **Figure 6**.

This figure shows significant cross-signaling between these various metabolic systems within the cell and potential inhibition or activation of one system by another. In some cases, there is mutual activation, such as between AMPK and SIRT or between PI3K/AKT (Phosphatidylinositol 3-kinase/protein kinase B), mTOR (mammalian target of rapamycin) and NF-κB. In other cases, there can be reciprocal inhibition between systems, such as between PI3K/AKT and AMPK. Finally, there can also be unidirectional inhibition or activation between various signaling pathways.

AMPK may represent the molecular link between these diverse signaling systems and the diet. This control is possible since AMPK is an evolutionarily conserved energy sensor that controls metabolism. In essence, AMPK becomes the checkpoint for metabolic control that links diet to other intracellular signaling systems.

However, one can only routinely monitor the blood, not the cell's interior. This inaccessibility of direct measurement of AMPK is why constant monitoring of the blood markers described above provides an easily obtained insight into AMPK activity. In

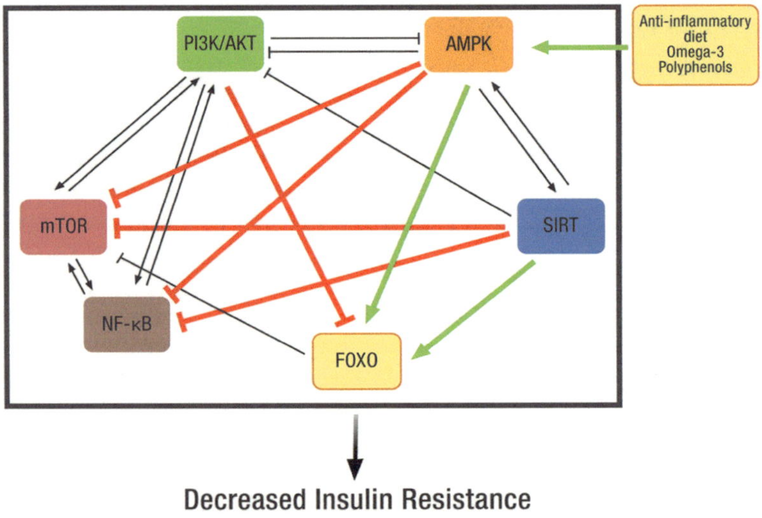

Figure 6.
Effect of dietary activation of AMPK on various regulatory proteins and gene transcription factors. Abbreviations: AMPK, 5′ adenosine monophosphate-activated protein kinase; FOXO, Forkhead box transcription factors class O; mTOR, mammalian target of rapamycin; NF-κB, nuclear factor kappa-B; Omega-3 PUFAs, Omega-3 polyunsaturated fatty acids; PI3K/AKT, phosphatidylinositol 3-kinase/AKT (protein kinase B); SIRT, Sirtuins. Green lines = activation; red lines = inhibition; black lines = mutual activation or mutual inhibition.

doing so, it may be possible to maintain these other internal cellular signaling pathways within their optimal operating parameters that are personalized to the subject.

The goal is to have AMPK able to respond dynamically to changing conditions in the cell. For example, there will be times when inflammation must be up-regulated but then returned to a quiescent state to maintain homeostasis. This molecular resilience requires keeping AMPK activity within discrete operating boundaries determined from surrogate markers in the blood. As pointed out above, each of these surrogate markers is under robust dietary control.

On the other hand, if AMPK activity is significantly inhibited, this leads to the over-expression of pro-inflammatory signaling systems shown in **Figure 6**. One of the linked systems that would increase with a decrease in AMPK activity is represented by the activation of NF-κB. Increased NF-κB activity is associated with increased inflammatory state related to cardiovascular disease [123] and cancer [124]. Likewise, reduced activity of AMPK would lead to potentially excessive activity of mTOR and PI3K/AKT signaling pathways associated with cancer [125, 126].

How the activity of AMPK acts as the intracellular central hub linking various other cellular signaling systems is described in more detail in the following paragraphs.

8.1 NF-κB signaling pathway

One of the primary benefits of activating AMPK is the inhibition of NF-κB, thus reducing pro-inflammatory cytokine and eicosanoid formation. The lowering of inflammation is achieved through several routes orchestrated by AMPK [60, 127]. One pathway is inhibiting NF-κB by the direct activation of AMPK [127]. Another pathway is activating sirtuin 1 (SIRT1) by increasing NAD^+ levels [128]. AMPK activates the rate-limiting enzyme in the NAD^+ salvage pathway that provides the necessary NAD^+ to enable SIRT1 to deacetylate the p65 Lys310 component of NF-κB to prevent its binding to the cell's DNA that is required to express inflammatory mediators [129].

Additional AMPK-mediated pathways that inhibit NF-κB activity include the activation of the Peroxisome proliferator-activated receptor-gamma coactivator 1-alpha (PGC-1α) [130] and the phosphorylation of Forkhead box transcription factors class O (FOXO) [127].

8.2 mTOR signaling pathway

Activation of AMPK is the primary inhibitor of mTOR. At the molecular level, mTOR inhibition is due to phosphorylation of the raptor component of mTORC1 and TSC2 [131]. In addition, the association of increased SIRT1 activity with mTOR inhibition [132] can be induced by the AMPK's activation of the rate-eliminating enzyme of the NAD+ salvage pathway [128]. On the other hand, any increase in AKT activity will up-regulate mTOR, which activates NF-κB [133].

8.3 PI3K/AKT signaling pathway

The PI3K/AKT signaling pathway is activated by insulin and results in cellular growth activation [134]. If the PI3K/AKT signaling pathway is overactive, this will inhibit the activity of AMPK [135, 136]. On the other hand, any increase in AMPK activation will inhibit AKT activity [135, 136].

Therefore, the inhibition of AMPK and FOXO activity by AKT can be reduced by dietary activation of AMPK. PI3K activity is reduced at the most basic level by lowering blood insulin levels following an anti-inflammatory calorie-restricted diet. The reduction of PI3K stimulation by insulin leads to decreased activation of AKT. Long-term studies using the previously described anti-inflammatory calorie-restricted diet have demonstrated success in the long-term management of type 2 diabetes mellitus [81, 84].

8.4 FOXO signaling pathway

The FOXO family of gene transcription factors consist of FOXO1, FOXO3, FOXO4, and FOXO6. The FOXO family is vital in controlling cellular senescence, stem cell maintenance, and lifespan in animal models [137]. FOXO upregulation can be achieved either by phosphorylation via AMPK or deacetylation by SIRT2 [138, 139]. In addition to the direct effect of AMPK activation on FOXO, any increase in AMPK activity will increase the activity of the rate-limiting enzyme (NAMPT) in the synthesis of NAD^+, thereby activating SIRT, which also increases FOXO activity [140].

An indirect route to activate FOXO is via the AMPK-induced inhibition of AKT [138]. On the other hand, any upregulation of AKT by a deficit in AMPK activity will reduce FOXO activity [141–143]. This central role of AMPK in FOXO activation may explain why activation of AMPK has been hypothesized to control the aging process [144].

Another inflammatory pathway that can be modulated by AMPK is JAK-STAT (Janus kinase-signal transducer and activator of transcription) signaling pathway, which mediates cytokine signaling [145].

Considering the complexity of these interactions with cellular signaling mechanisms in the cell, optimizing AMPK activity may have a far greater potential to bring a cell back to homeostasis than any current or proposed potential drug therapies. Furthermore, the dietary interventions described above have a potential therapeutic index that is significantly higher in reducing insulin resistance compared to any drug therapy.

9. Conclusions

We hypothesize that the ability to reduce severe insulin resistance caused by lipodystrophy and other conditions associated with insulin resistance may be achieved by increasing AMPK activity. Our hypothesis is based on the ability of AMPK to modulate internal cellular signaling through systems-based biology. While there is no single specific nutrient to optimize the body's internal capacity to alleviate insulin resistance, an appropriate combination of dietary interventions can alter signaling pathways that can lead to the molecular goal of increasing AMPK activity.

This concept of requiring a defined variety of multiple dietary interventions to achieve the appropriate activation of AMPK is no different from using various combinations of chemotherapeutic drugs to treat cancer. However, unlike numerous combination drug therapies used for cancer treatment, each dietary intervention described earlier can be easily modulated on a personalized basis using the clinical markers described earlier.

In conclusion, understanding the complex interaction of highly defined dietary interventions that result in the activation of AMPK may provide a new comprehensive nutritional strategy to treat insulin resistance induced by lipodystrophy. The same dietary technology is also applicable to many other chronic conditions associated with insulin resistance. Furthermore, the dietary approach we have outlined can be optimized individually using validated blood markers to orchestrate various internal cellular signaling systems. Using such blood markers to titrate each dietary component that impacts activation of AMPK to their appropriate ranges moves precision nutrition into the realm of personalized medicine.

Acknowledgements

This study was supported by the Inflammation Research Foundation, Peabody, MA, USA.

Author contributions

BS and AKS wrote the paper.

Conflicts of interest

BS and AKS are employed by Zone Labs, Inc., a medical foods company.

Author details

Barry Sears* and Asish K. Saha
Inflammation Research Foundation, Peabody, MA, USA

*Address all correspondence to: bsears@drsears.com

References

[1] Longo M, Zatterale F, Naderi J, Parrillo L, Formisano P, Raciti GA, et al. Adipose tissue dysfunction as determinant of obesity-associated metabolic complications. International Journal of Molecular Sciences. 2019;**20**:2358. DOI: 10.3390/ijms20092358

[2] Yazıcı D, Sezer H. Insulin resistance, obesity and lipotoxicity. Obesity and Lipotoxicity. 2017;**960**:277-304. DOI: 10.1007/978-3-319-48382-512

[3] Chan JL, Oral EA. Clinical classification and treatment of congenital and acquired lipodystrophy. Endocrine Practice. 2010;**16**:310-323

[4] Garg A. Clinical review#: Lipodystrophies: Genetic and acquired body fat disorders. The Journal of Clinical Endocrinology and Metabolism. 2010;**16**:310-323. DOI: 10.4158/EP09154.RA

[5] Angelidi AM, Filippaios A, Mantzoros CS. Severe insulin resistance syndromes. The Journal of Clinical Investigation. 2021;**131**:e142245. DOI: 10.1172/JCI142245

[6] Obradovic M, Sudar-Milovanovic E, Soskic S, Essack M, Arya S, Stewart AJ, et al. Leptin and obesity: Role and clinical implication. Frontiers in Endocrinology (Lausanne). 2021;**12**:585887. DOI: 10.3389/fendo.2021.585887

[7] Koethe JR, Lagathu C, Lake JE, Domingo P, Calmy A, Falutz J, et al. HIV and antiretroviral therapy-related fat alterations. Nature Reviews Disease Primers. 2020;**6**(48). DOI: 10.1038/s41572-020-0181-1

[8] Araújo-Vilar D, Santini F. Diagnosis and treatment of lipodystrophy: A step-by-step approach. Journal of Endocrinological Investigation. 2019;**42**:61-73. DOI: 10.1007/s40618-018-0887-z

[9] Gentile S, Strollo F, Ceriello A. Lipodystrophy in insulin-treated subjects and other injection-site skin reactions: Are we sure everything is clear? Diabetes Therapy. 2016;**7**:401-409. DOI: 10.1007/s13300-016-0187-6

[10] DeFronzo RA. Insulin resistance, lipotoxicity, type 2 diabetes and atherosclerosis: The missing links. Diabetologia. 2010;**53**:1270-1287. DOI: 10.1007/s00125-010-1684-1

[11] Belsham DD, Dalvi PS. Insulin signalling in hypothalamic neurons. Journal of Neuroendocrinology. 2020;**33**:e12919. DOI: 10.1111/jne.12919

[12] Meex RCR, Blaak EE, van Loon LJC. Lipotoxicity plays a key role in the development of both insulin resistance and muscle atrophy in patients with type 2 diabetes. Obesity Reviews. 2019;**20**:1205-1217. DOI: 10.1111/obr.12862

[13] Lim K, Haider A, Adams C, Sleigh A, Savage DB. Lipodistrophy: A paradigm for understanding the consequences of "overloading" adipose tissue. Physiological Reviews. 2021;**101**:907-993. DOI: 10.1152/physrev.00032.2020

[14] Himsworth HP. Diabetes mellitus: Its differentiation into insulin-sensitive and insulin-insensitive types. Lancet. 1936;**227**:127-130. DOI: 10.1016/S0140-6736(01)36134-2

[15] Reaven GM. Banting lecture 1988. Role of insulin resistance in human disease. Diabetes. 1988;**37**:1595-1607. DOI: 10.2337/diabetes.37.12.1595

[16] Yaribeygi H, Farrokhi FR, Butler AE, Sahebkar A. Insulin resistance: Review of the underlying molecular mechanisms. Journal of Cellular Physiology. 2019;**234**: 8152-8161. DOI: 10.1002/jcp.27603

[17] Petersen MC, Shulman GI. Mechanisms of insulin action and insulin resistance. Physiological Reviews. 2018;**98**:2133-2223. DOI: 10.1152/physrev.00063.2017

[18] Hotamisligil GS. Inflammation and metabolic disorders. Nature. 2006;**444**:860-867. DOI: 10.1038/nature05485

[19] Chen L, Chen R, Wang H, Liang F. Mechanisms linking inflammation to insulin resistance. International Journal of Endocrinology. 2015;**2015**:508409. DOI: 10.1155/2015/508409

[20] Hotamisligil GS. Foundations of immunometabolism and implications for metabolic health and disease. Immunity. 2017;**47**:406-420. DOI: 10.1016/j.immuni.2017.08.009

[21] Lee YS, Olefsky J. Chronic tissue inflammation and metabolic disease. Genes & Development. 2021;**35**:307-328. DOI: 10.1101/gad.346312.120

[22] Singh B, Saxena A. Surrogate markers of insulin resistance: A review. World Journal of Diabetes. 2010;**1**:36-47. DOI: 10.4239/wjd.v1.i2.36

[23] Randle PJ, Garland PB, Hales CN, Newsholme EA. The glucose fatty-acid cycle. Its role in insulin sensitivity and the metabolic disturbances of diabetes mellitus. The Lancet. 1963;**281**(7285):785-789. DOI: 10.1016/s0140-6736(63)91500-9

[24] Boden G, Chen X, Ruiz J, White JV, Rossetti L. Mechanisms of fatty acid-induced inhibition of glucose uptake. The Journal of Clinical Investigation. 1994;**93**:2438-2446. DOI: 10.1172/JCI117252

[25] Shulman GI, Rothman DL, Jue T, Stein P, DeFronzo RA, Shulman RG. Quantitation of muscle glycogen synthesis in normal subjects and subjects with non-insulin-dependent diabetes by 13C nuclear magnetic resonance spectroscopy. The New England Journal of Medicine. 1990;**322**:223-228. DOI: 10.1056/NEJM199001253220403

[26] Reali F, Morine MJ, Kahramanoğulları O, Raichur S, Schneider HC, Crowther D, et al. Mechanistic interplay between ceramide and insulin resistance. Scientific Reports. 2017;**7**:41231. DOI: 10.1038/srep41231

[27] Hue L, Taegtmeyer H. The Randle cycle revisited: A new head for an old hat. American Journal of Physiology. Endocrinology and Metabolism. 2009;**297**:E578-E591. DOI: 10.1152/ajpendo.00093.2009

[28] Savage DB, Petersen KF, Shulman GI. Mechanisms of insulin resistance in humans and possible links with inflammation. Hypertension. 2005;**45**:828-833. DOI: 10.1161/01.HYP.0000163475.04421.e4

[29] Hotamisligil GS, Shargill NS, Spiegelman BM. Adipose expression of tumor necrosis factor-alpha: Direct role in obesity-linked insulin resistance. Science. 1993;**259**:87-91. DOI: 10.1126/science.7678183

[30] Hotamisligil GS. Inflammatory pathways and insulin action. International Journal of Obesity and Related Metabolic Disorders. 2003;**27**(3):S53-S55. DOI: 10.1038/sj.ijo.0802502

[31] Kanety H, Feinstein R, Papa MZ, Hemi R, Karasik A. Tumor necrosis

factor alpha-induced phosphorylation of insulin receptor substrate-1 (IRS-1). Possible mechanism for suppression of insulin-stimulated tyrosine phosphorylation of IRS-1. The Journal of Biological Chemistry. 1995;**270**:23780-23784. DOI: 10.1074/jbc.270.40.23780

[32] Li B, Leung JCK, Chan LYY, Yiu WH, Tang SCW. A global perspective on the crosstalk between saturated fatty acids and toll-like receptor 4 in the etiology of inflammation and insulin resistance. Progress in Lipid Research. 2020;**77**:101020. DOI: 10.1016/j.plipres.2019.101020

[33] Hundal RS, Petersen KF, Mayerson AB, Randhawa PS, Inzucchi S, Shoelson SE, et al. Mechanism by which high-dose aspirin improves glucose metabolism in type 2 diabetes. The Journal of Clinical Investigation. 2002;**109**:1321-1326. DOI: 10.1172/JCI14955

[34] Shoelson SE, Lee J, Goldfine AB. Inflammation and insulin resistance. The Journal of Clinical Investigation. 2006;**116**:1793-1801. DOI: 10.1172/JCI29069

[35] Goldfine AB, Fonseca V, Jablonski KA, Chen YD, Tipton L, Staten MA, et al. Salicylate (salsalate) in patients with type 2 diabetes: A randomized trial. Targeting inflammation using Salsalate in type 2 diabetes study team. Annals of Internal Medicine. 2013;**159**:1-12. DOI: 10.7326/0003-4819-159-1-201307020-00003

[36] Hirosumi J, Tuncman G, Chang L, Görgün CZ, Uysal KT, Maeda K, et al. A central role for JNK in obesity and insulin resistance. Nature. 2002;**420**:333-336. DOI: 10.1038/nature01137

[37] Johanns M, Lai Y-C, Hsu M-F, Jacobs R, Vertommen D, Sande JV, et al. AMPK antagonizes hepatic glucagon-stimulated cyclic AMP signalling via phosphorylation-induced activation of cyclic nucleotide phosphodiesterase 4B. Nature Communications. 2016;**7**:10856. DOI: 10.1038/ncomms10856

[38] Sancar G, Liu S, Gasser E, Alvarez JG, Moutos C, Kim K, et al. FGF1 and insulin control lipolysis by convergent pathways. Cell Metabolism. 2022;**34**:171-183.e6. DOI: 10.1016/j.cmet.2021.12.004

[39] Fryer LGD, Parbu-Patel A, Carling D. The anti-diabetic drugs rosiglitazone and metformin stimulate AMP-activated protein kinase through distinct signaling pathways. The Journal of Biological Chemistry. 2002;**277**:25226-25232. DOI: 10.1074/jbc.M202489200

[40] Saha AK, Avilucea PR, Ye JM, Assifi MM, Kraegen EW, Ruderman NB. Pioglitazone treatment activates AMP-activated protein kinase in rat liver and adipose tissue in vivo. Biochemical and Biophysical Research Communications. 2004;**314**:580-585. DOI: 10.1016/j.bbrc.2003.12.120

[41] LeBrasseur NK, Kelly M, Tsao TS, Farmer SR, Saha AK, Ruderman NB, et al. Thiazolidinediones can rapidly activate AMP-activated protein kinase in mammalian tissues. American Journal of Physiology. Endocrinology and Metabolism. 2006;**291**:E175-E181. DOI: 10.1152/ajpendo.00453.2005

[42] Zhao Z, Lee YJ, Kim SK, Kim HZ, Shim WS, Ahn CW, et al. Rosiglitazone and fenofibrate improve insulin sensitivity of pre-diabetic OLETF rats by reducing malonyl-CoA levels in the liver and skeletal muscle. Life Sciences. 2009;**84**:688-695. DOI: 10.1016/j.lfs.2009.02.021

[43] Day EA, Ford RJ, Steinberg GR. AMPK as a therapeutic target for

treating metabolic diseases. Trends in Endocrinology & Metabolism. 2017;**28**:545-560. DOI: 10.1016/j.tem.2017.05.004

[44] Saha AK, Xu XJ, Balon TW, Brandon A, Kraegen EW, Ruderman NB. Insulin resistance due to nutrient excess: Is it a consequence of AMPK downregulation? Cell Cycle. 2011;**10**:3447-3451. DOI: 10.4161/cc.10.20.17886

[45] Ruderman NB, Carling D, Prentki M, Cacicedo JM. AMPK insulin resistance, and the metabolic syndrome. The Journal of Clinical Investigation. 2013;**123**:2764-2772. DOI: 10.1172/JCI67227

[46] Lyons CL, Roche HM. Nutritional modulation of AMPK-impact upon metabolic-inflammation. International Journal of Molecular Sciences. 2018;**19**:3092. DOI: 10.3390/ijms19103092

[47] Jeon SM. Regulation and function of AMPK in physiology and diseases. Experimental & Molecular Medicine. 2016;**48**:e245. DOI: 10.1038/emm.2016.81

[48] Smith BK, Marcinko K, Desjardins EM, Lally JS, Ford RJ, Steinberg GR. Treatment of non-alcoholic fatty liver disease: Role of AMPK. American Journal of Physiology. Endocrinology and Metabolism. 2016;**311**:E730-E740. DOI: 10.1152/ajpendo.00225.2016

[49] Desjardins EM, Steinberg GR. Emerging role of AMPK in brown and beige adipose tissue (BAT): Implications for obesity, insulin resistance, and type 2 diabetes. Current Diabetes Reports. 2018;**18**:80. DOI: 10.1007/s11892-018-1049-6

[50] Wang F, Han L, Hu D. Fasting insulin, insulin resistance and risk of hypertension in the general population: A meta-analysis. Clinica Chimica Acta. 2017;**464**:57-63. DOI: 10.1016/j.cca.2016.11.009

[51] Laakso M, Kuusisto J. Insulin resistance and hyperglycaemia in cardiovascular disease development. Nature Reviews Endocrinology. 2014;**10**:293-302. DOI: 10.1038/nrendo.2014.29

[52] Diamanti-Kandarakis E, Dunaif A. Insulin resistance and the polycystic ovary syndrome revisited: An update on mechanisms and implications. Endocrine Reviews. 2012;**33**:981-1030. DOI: 10.1210/er.2011-1034

[53] Spoto B, Pisano A, Zoccali C. Insulin resistance in chronic kidney disease: A systematic review. American Journal of Physiology. Renal Physiology. 2016;**311**:F1087-F1108. DOI: 10.1152/ajprenal.00340.2016

[54] Arcidiacono B, Iiritano S, Nocera A, Possidente K, Nevolo MT, Ventura V, et al. Insulin resistance and cancer risk: An overview of the pathogenetic mechanisms. Experimental Diabetes Research. 2012;**2012**:789174. DOI: 10.1155/2012/789174

[55] Leonard BE, Wegener G. Inflammation, insulin resistance and neuroprogression in depression. Acta Neuropsychiatrica. 2020;**32**:1-9. DOI: 10.1017/neu.2019.17

[56] Hölscher C. Brain insulin resistance: Role in neurodegenerative disease and potential for targeting. Expert Opinion on Investigational Drugs. 2020;**29**: 333-348. DOI: 10.1080/13543784.2020.1738383

[57] Sears B, Perry M, Saha AK. Dietary technologies to optimize healing from injury-induced inflammation. Antiinflammory & Antiallergy Agents in Medicinal Chemistry. 2021;**20**:

123-131. DOI: 10.2174/187152301966620
0512114210

[58] Sears B, Saha AK. Dietary control of inflammation and resolution. Frontiers in Nutrition. 2021;**8**. DOI: 10.3389/fnut.2021.709435

[59] Nunes AK, Rapôso C, Rocha SW, Barbosa KP, Luna RL, da Cruz-Höfling MA, et al. Involvement of AMPK, IKβα-NFκB and eNOS in the sildenafil anti-inflammatory mechanism in a demyelination model. Brain Research. 2015;**1627**:119-133. DOI: 10.1016/j.brainres.2015.09.008

[60] Salminen A, Hyttinen JMT, Kaamiranta K. AMP-activated protein kinase inhibits NF-κB signaling and inflammation: Impact on healthspan and lifespan. Journal of Molecular Medicine (Berlin). 2011;**89**:667-676. DOI: 10.1007/s00109-011-0748-0

[61] Farias MR, Domenech JF, Serra D, Herrero L, Infantes DS. White adipose tissue dysfunction in obesity and aging. Biochemical Pharmacology. 2021;**192**:114723. DOI: 10.1016/j.bcp.2021.114723

[62] Xu XJ, Apovian C, Hess D, Carmine B, Saha A, Ruderman N. Improved insulin sensitivity 3 months after RYGB surgery is associated with increased subcutaneous adipose tissue AMPK activity and decreased oxidative stress. Diabetes. 2015;**64**:3155-3159. DOI: 10.2337/db14-1765

[63] Gauthier MS, O'Brien EL, Bigornia S, Mott M, Cacicedo JM, Xu XJ, et al. Decreased AMP-activated protein kinase activity is associated with increased inflammation in visceral adipose tissue and with whole-body insulin resistance in morbidly obese humans. Biochemical and Biophysical Research Communications. 2010;**404**(1):382-387. DOI: 10.1016/j.bbrc.2010.11.127

[64] Rena G, Hardie DG, Pearson ER. The mechanisms of action of metformin. Diabetologia. 2017;**60**:1577-1585. DOI: 10.1007/s00125-017-4342-z

[65] Foretz M, Guigas B, Viollet B. Understanding the glucoregulatory mechanisms of metformin in type 2 diabetes mellitus. Nature Reviews. Endocrinology. 2019;**15**:569-589. DOI: 10.1038/s41574-019-0242-2

[66] Hawley SA, Ford RJ, Smith BK, Gowans GJ, Mancini SJ, Pitt RD, et al. The Na+/glucose cotransporter inhibitor canagliflozin activates AMPK by inhibiting mitochondrial function and increasing cellular AMP levels. Diabetes. 2016;**65**:2784-2794. DOI: 10.2337/db16-0058

[67] Hwang HJ, Jung TW, Kim BH, Hong HC, Seo JA, Kim SG, et al. A dipeptidyl peptidase-IV inhibitor improves hepatic steatosis and insulin resistance by AMPK-dependent and JNK-dependent inhibition of LECT2 expression. Biochemical Pharmacology. 2015;**98**:157-166. DOI: 10.1016/j.bcp.2015.08.098

[68] Zhou JY, Poudel A, Welchko R, Mekala N, Chandramani-Shivalingappa P, Rosca MG, et al. Liraglutide improves insulin sensitivity in high fat diet induced diabetic mice through multiple pathways. European Journal of Pharmacology. 2019;**861**:172594. DOI: 10.1016/j.ejphar.2019.172594

[69] Cantó C, Auwerx J. Calorie restriction: Is AMPK as a key sensor and effector? Physiology (Bethesda). 2011;**26**:214-224. DOI: 10.1152/physiol.00010.2011

[70] Kraus WE, Bhapkar M, Huffman KM, Pieper CF, Krupa Das S,

Redman LM, et al. 2 years of calorie restriction and cardiometabolic risk (CALERIE): Exploratory outcomes of a multicentre, phase 2, randomised controlled trial. The Lancet Diabetes and Endocrinology. 2019;7:673-683. DOI: 10.1016/S2213-8587(19)30151-2

[71] Ludwig DS, Majzoub JA, Al-Zahrani A, Dallal GE, Blanco I, Roberts SB. High glycemic index foods, overeating, and obesity. Pediatrics. 1999;**103**:E26. DOI: 10.1542/peds.103.3.e26

[72] Veldhorst M, Smeets A, Soenen S, Hochstenbach-Waelen A, Hursel R, Diepvens K, et al. Protein-induced satiety: Effects and mechanisms of different proteins. Physiology & Behavior. 2008;**94**:300-307. DOI: 10.1016/j.physbeh.2008.01.003

[73] Shukla AP, Andono J, Touhamy SH, Casper A, Iliescu RG, Mauer E, et al. Carbohydrate-last meal pattern lowers postprandial glucose and insulin excursions in type 2 diabetes. BMJ Open Diabetes Research & Care. 2017;5:e000440. DOI: 10.1136/bmjdrc-2017-000440

[74] Simpson SJ, Raubenheimer D. Obesity: The protein leverage hypothesis. Obesity Reviews. 2005;**6**:133-142. DOI: 10.1111/j.1467-789X.2005.00178.x

[75] Sears B. The Zone. NY: Harper Collins; 1995

[76] Brenner RR. Hormonal modulation of delta6 and delta5 desaturases: Case of diabetes. Prostaglandins, Leukotrienes, and Essential Fatty Acids. 2003;**68**:151-162. DOI: 10.1016/s0952-3278(02)00265-x

[77] Zhou J, Martin RJ, Tulley RT, Raggio AM, McCutcheon KL, Shen L, et al. Dietary resistant starch upregulates total GLP-1 and PYY in a sustained day-long manner through fermentation in rodents. American Journal of Physiology. Endocrinology and Metabolism. 2008;**295**:E1160-E1166. DOI: 10.1152/ajpendo.90637.2008

[78] Schaeffler A, Gross P, Buettner R, Bollheimer C, Buechler C, Neumeier M, et al. Fatty acid-induced induction of toll-like receptor-4/nuclear factor-kappaB pathway in adipocytes links nutritional signalling with innate immunity. Immunology. 2009;**126**:233-245. DOI: 10.1111/j.1365-2567.2008.02892.x

[79] Markovic TP, Jenkins AB, Campbell LV, Furler SM, Kraegen EW, Chisholm DJ. The determinants of glycemic responses to diet restriction and weight loss in obesity and NIDDM. Diabetes Care. 1998;**21**:687-694. DOI: 10.2337/diacare.21.5.687

[80] Gannon MC, Nuttall FQ, Saeed A, Jordan K, Hoover H. An increase in dietary protein improves the blood glucose response in persons with type 2 diabetes. The American Journal of Clinical Nutrition. 2003;**78**:734-741. DOI: 10.1093/ajcn/78.4.734

[81] Hamdy O, Carver C. The why WAIT program: Improving clinical outcomes through weight management in type 2 diabetes. Current Diabetes Reports. 2008;**8**:413-420. DOI: 10.1007/s11892-008-0071-5

[82] Mottalib A, Sakr M, Shehabeldin M, Hamdy O. Diabetes remission after nonsurgical intensive lifestyle intervention in obese patients with type 2 diabetes. Journal Diabetes Research. 2015;**2015**:468704. DOI: 10.1155/2015/468704

[83] Markova M, Pivovarova O, Hornemann S, Sucher S, Frahnow T, Wegner K, et al. Isocaloric diets high

in animal or plant protein reduce liver fat and inflammation in individuals with type 2 diabetes. Gastroenterology. 2017;**152**:571-585. DOI: 10.1053/j.gastro.2016.10.007

[84] Hamdy O, Mottalib A, Morsi A, El-Sayed N, Goebel-Fabbri A, Arathuzik G, et al. Long-term effect of intensive lifestyle intervention on cardiovascular risk factors in patients with diabetes in real-world clinical practice: A 5-year longitudinal study. BMJ Open Diabetes Research & Care. 2017;**5**:e000259. DOI: 10.1136/bmjdrc-2016-000259

[85] Liu K, Wang B, Zhou R, Lang HD, Ran L, Wang J, et al. Effect of combined use of a low-carbohydrate, high-protein diet with omega-3 polyunsaturated fatty acid supplementation on glycemic control in newly diagnosed type 2 diabetes: A randomized, double-blind, parallel-controlled trial. The American Journal of Clinical Nutrition. 2018;**108**:256-265. DOI: 10.1093/ajcn/nqy120

[86] Samkani A, Skytte MJ, Kandel D, Kjaer S, Astrup A, Deacon CF, et al. A carbohydrate-reduced high-protein diet acutely decreases postprandial and diurnal glucose excursions in type 2 diabetes patients. The British Journal of Nutrition. 2018;**119**:910-917. DOI: 10.1017/S0007114518000521

[87] Coussa A, Bassil M, Gougeon R, Marliss EB, Morais JA. Glucose and protein metabolic responses to an energy- but not protein- restricted diet in type 2 diabetes. Diabetes, Obesity & Metabolism. 2020;**22**:1278-1285. DOI: 10.1111/dom.14026

[88] Stentz FB, Mikhael A, Kineish O, Christman J, Sands C. High protein diet leads to prediabetes remission and positive changes in incretins and cardiovascular risk factors. Nutrition, Metabolism, and Cardiovascular Diseases. 2021;**31**:1227-1237. DOI: 10.1016/j.numecd.2020.11.027

[89] Marra M, Sammarco R, De Lorenzo A, Iellamo F, Siervo M, Pietrobelli A, et al. Assessment of body composition in health and disease using bioelectrical impedance analysis (BIA) and dual energy X-ray absorptiometry (DXA): A critical overview. Contrast Media & Molecular Imaging. 2010;**2019**:3548284. DOI: 10.1155/2019/3548284 eCollection 2019

[90] Meeuwsen S, Horgan GW, Elia M. The relationship between BMI and percent body fat, measured by bioelectrical impedance, in a large adult sample is curvilinear and influenced by age and sex. Clinical Nutrition. 2010;**29**:560-566. DOI: 10.1016/j.clnu.2009.12.011

[91] Foretz M, Even PC, Viollet B. AMPK activation reduces hepatic lipid content by increasing fat oxidation in vivo. International Journal of Molecular Sciences. 2018;**19**:2826. DOI: 10.3390/ijms19092826

[92] Lin SC, Hardie DG. AMPK: Sensing glucose as well as cellular energy status. Cell Metabolism. 2018;**27**:299-313. DOI: 10.1016/j.cmet.2017.10.009

[93] Saha AK, Xu XJ, Lawson E, Deoliveira R, Brandon AE, Kraegen EW, et al. Downregulation of AMPK accompanies leucine- and glucose-induced increases in protein synthesis and insulin resistance in rat skeletal muscle. Diabetes. 2010;**59**:2426-2434. DOI: 10.2337/db09-1870

[94] Hosseini Z, Marinello M, Decker C, Sansbury BE, Sadhu S, Gerlach BD, et al. Resolvin D1 enhances necroptotic cell clearance through promoting

macrophage fatty acid oxidation and oxidative phosphorylation. Arteriosclerosis, Thrombosis, and Vascular Biology. 2021;**41**:1062-1075. DOI: 10.1161/ATVBAHA.120.315758

[95] Jung TW, Kim HC, Abd El-Aty AM, Jeong JH. Protectin DX ameliorates palmitate- or high-fat diet-induced insulin resistance and inflammation through an AMPK-PPARalpha-dependent pathway in mice. Scientific Reports. 2017;**7**:1397. DOI: 10.1038/s41598-017-01603-9

[96] Recchiuti A, Isopi E, Romano M, Mattoscio D. Roles of specialized pro-resolving lipid mediators in autophagy and inflammation. International Journal of Molecular Sciences. 2020;**21**(18):6637. DOI: 10.3390/ijms21186637

[97] Cory H, Passarelli S, Szeto J, Tamez M, Mattei J. The role of polyphenols in human health and food systems: A mini-review. Frontiers in Nutrition. 2018;**5**:87. DOI: 10.3389/fnut.2018.00087

[98] Nunes RD, Ventura-Martins GM, Moretti DM, Medeiros-Castro P, Rocha-Santos C, et al. Polyphenol-rich diets exacerbate AMPK-mediated autophagy, decreasing proliferation of mosquito midgut microbiota, and extending vector lifespan. PLoS Neglected Tropical Diseases. 2016;**10**(10):e0005034. DOI: 10.1371/journal.pntd.0005034

[99] Hou X, Xu S, Maitland-Toolan KA, Sato K, Jiang B, Ido Y, et al. SIRT1 regulates hepatocyte lipid metabolism through activating AMP-activated protein kinase. The Journal of Biological Chemistry. 2008;**283**:20015-20026. DOI: doi.org/10.1074/jbc.M802187200

[100] Imai SI, Guarente L. It takes two to tango: NAD(+) and sirtuins in aging/longevity control. NPJ Aging and Mechanisms of Disease. 2016;**2**:16017. DOI: 10.1038/npjamd.2016.17

[101] Rothgiesser KM, Erener S, Waibel S, Lüscher B, Hottiger MO. SIRT2 regulates NF-κB dependent gene expression through deacetylation of p65 Lys310. Journal of Cell Science. 2010;**123**(24):4251-4258. DOI: 10.1242/jcs.073783

[102] Matzinger M, Fischhuber K, Pölöske D, Mechtler K, Heiss EH. AMPK leads to phosphorylation of the transcription factor Nrf2, tuning transactivation of selected target genes. Redox Biology. 2020;**29**:101393. DOI: 10.1016/j.redox.2019.101393

[103] Schön C, Wacker R, Micka A, Steudle J, Lang S, Bonnländer B. Bioavailability study of maqui berry extract in healthy subjects. Nutrients. 2018;**10**:1720. DOI: 10.3390/nu10111720

[104] Davinelli S, Bertoglio JC, Zarrelli A, Pina R, Scapagnini G. A randomized clinical trial evaluating the efficacy of an anthocyanin-maqui berry extract (Delphinol®) on oxidative stress biomarkers. Journal of the American College of Nutrition. 2015;**34**:28-33. DOI: 10.1080/07315724.2015.1080108

[105] McLaughlin T, Allison G, Abbasi F, Lamendola C, Reaven GM. Prevalence of insulin resistance and associated cardiovascular disease risk factors among normal weight, overweight, and obese individuals. Metabolism. 2004;**53**:495-499. DOI: 10.1016/j.metabol.2003.10.032

[106] Gonzalez-Chavez A, Simental-Mendia LE, Elizondo-Argueta S. Elevated triglycerides/HDL-cholesterol ratio associated with insulin resistance. Cirugia y Cirujanos. 2011;**79**:126-131 PMID: 21631973

[107] Pantoja-Torres B, Toro-Huamanchumo CJ, Urrunaga-Pastor D, Guarnizo-Poma M, Lazaro-Alcantara H, Paico-Palacios S, et al. High triglyceride to HDL-cholesterol ratio is associated with insulin resistance in normal-weight healthy adults. Diabetes & Metabolic Syndrome. 2019;**13**:382-388. DOI: 10.1016/j.dsx.2018.10.006

[108] Murguia-RomeroM,Jimenez-FloresJR, Sigrist-FloresSC,Espinoza-CamachoMA, Jiménez-Morales M, Pina E, et al. Plasma triglyceride/HDLcholesterol ratio, insulin resistance, and cardiometabolic risk in young adults. Journal of Lipid Research. 2013;**54**:2795-2799. DOI: 10.1194/jlr.M040584

[109] Fan X, Liu EY, Hoffman VP, Potts AJ, Sharma B, Henderson DC. Triglyceride/high-density lipoprotein cholesterol ratio: A surrogate to predict insulin resistance and low-density lipoprotein cholesterol particle size in nondiabetic patients with schizophrenia. The Journal of Clinical Psychiatry. 2011;**72**:806-812. DOI: 10.4088/JCP.09m05107yel

[110] Quispe R, Martin SS, Jones SR. Triglycerides to high-density lipoprotein-cholesterol ratio, glycemic control and cardiovascular risk in obese patients with type 2 diabetes. Current Opinion in Endocrinology, Diabetes and Obesity. 2016;**23**:150-156. DOI: 10.1097/MED.0000000000000241

[111] Salazar MR, Carbajal HA, Espeche WG, Aizpurúa M, Marillet AG, Leiva Sisnieguez CE. Use of the triglyceride/high-density lipoprotein cholesterol ratio to identify cardiometabolic risk: Impact of obesity? Journal of Investigative Medicine. 2017;**65**:323-327. DOI: 10.1136/jim-2016-000248

[112] Lind L, Ingelsson E, Arnlov J, Sundström J, Zethelius B, Reaven GM. Can the plasma concentration ratio of triglyceride/high-density lipoprotein cholesterol identify individuals at high risk of cardiovascular disease during 40-year follow-up? Metabolic Syndrome and Related Disorders. 2018;**16**:433-439. DOI: 10.1089/met.2018.0058

[113] Endres S, Ghorbani R, Kelley VE, Georgilis K, Lonnemann G, van der Meer JW, et al. The effect of dietary supplementation with n-3 polyunsaturated fatty acids on the synthesis of interleukin-1 and tumor necrosis factor by mononuclear cells. The New England Journal of Medicine. 1989;**320**:265-271. DOI: 10.1056/NEJM198902023200501

[114] Tan A, Sullenbarger B, Prakash R, McDaniel JC. Supplementation with eicosapentaenoic acid and docosahexaenoic acid reduces high levels of circulating pro-inflammatory cytokines in aging adults: A randomized, controlled study. Prostaglandins, Leukotrienes, and Essential Fatty Acids. 2018;**132**:23-29. DOI: 10.1016/j.plefa.2018.03.010

[115] Madison AA, Belury MA, Andridge R, Renna ME, Shrout MR, Malarkey WB, et al. Omega-3 supplementation and stress reactivity of cellular aging biomarkers. Molecular Psychiatry. 2021;**2021**:2. DOI: doi.org/10.1038/s41380-021-01077-2

[116] Harris WS, Pottala JV, Lacey SM, Vasan RG, Larson MG, Robins SJ. Clinical correlates and heritability of erythrocyte eicosapentaenoic and docosahexaenoic acid content in the Framingham heart study. Atherosclerosis. 2012;**225**:425-431. DOI: 10.1016/j.atherosclerosis.2012.05.030

[117] Harris WS, Pottala JV, Varvel SA, Borowski JJ, Ward JN, McConnell JP. Erythrocyte omega-3 fatty acids increase

and linoleic acid decreases with age: Observations from 160,000 patients. Prostaglandins, Leukotrienes and Essential Fatty Acids. 2013;**88**:257-263. DOI: 10.1016/j.plefa.2012.12.004

[118] Shan Luo S, Schooling CM, Wong ICK, Yeung SLA. Evaluating the impact of AMPK activation, a target of metformin, on risk of cardiovascular diseases and cancer in the UK biobank: A Mendelian randomisation study. Diabetologia. 2020;**63**:2349-2358. DOI: doi.org/10.1007/s00125-020-05243-z

[119] Miyagishima KJ, Sharma R, Nimmagadda M, Clore-Gronenborn K, Qureshy Z, Ortolan D, et al. AMPK modulation ameliorates dominant disease phenotypes of CTRP5 variant in retinal degeneration. Communications Biology. 2021;**4**:1360. DOI: 10.1038/s42003-021-02872-x

[120] Hołowko J, Michalczyk MM, Zając A, Czerwińska-Rogowska M, Ryterska K, Banaszczak M, et al. Six weeks of calorie restriction improves body composition and lipid profile in obese and overweight former athletes. Nutrients. 2019;**11**:1461. DOI: 10.3390/nu11071461

[121] Alvarado J, Schoenlau F, Leschot A, Salgad AM, Vigil PP. Delphinol® standardized maqui berry extract significantly lowers blood glucose and improves blood lipid profile in prediabetic individuals in three-month clinical trial. Panminerva Medica. 2016;**58**:1-6 PMID: 27820958

[122] de Castro GS, Calder PC. Non-alcoholic fatty liver disease and its treatment with n-3 polyunsaturated fatty acids. Clinical Nutrition. 2018;**37**:37-55. DOI: 10.1016/j.clnu.2017.01.006

[123] Kaptoge S, Seshasai SR, Gao P, Freitag DF, Butterworth AS, Borglykke A. Inflammatory cytokines and risk of coronary heart disease: New prospective study and updated meta-analysis. European Heart Journal. 2014;**35**:578-589. DOI: 10.1093/eurheartj/eht367

[124] Hoesel B, Schmid JA. The complexity of NF-kappaB signaling in inflammation and cancer. Molecular Cancer. 2013;**12**:86. DOI: 10.1186/1476-4598-12-86

[125] Mossmann D, Park S, Hall MN. mTOR signalling and cellular metabolism are mutual determinants in cancer. Nature Reviews. Cancer. 2018;**18**:744-757. DOI: 10.1038/s41568-018-0074-8

[126] Noorolyai S, Shajari N, Baghbani E, Sadreddini S, Baradaran B. The relation between PI3K/AKT signalling pathway and cancer. Gene. 2019;**698**:120-128. DOI: 10.1016/j.gene.2019.02.076

[127] Xiang HC, Lin LX, Hu XF, Zhu H, Li HP, Zhang RY, et al. AMPK activation attenuates inflammatory pain through inhibiting NF-κB activation and IL-1β expression. Journal of Neuroinflammation. 2019;**16**:34. DOI: 10.1186/s12974-019-1411-x

[128] Brandauer J, Vienberg SG, Andersen MA, Ringholm S, Risis S, Larsen PS, et al. AMP-activated protein kinase regulates nicotinamide phosphoribosyl ltransferase expression in skeletal muscle. The Journal of Physiology. 2011;**591**:5207-5220. DOI: 10.1113/jphysiol.2013.259515

[129] Kauppinen A, Suuronen T, Ojala J, Kaarniranta K, Salminen A. Antagonistic crosstalk between NF-kappaB and SIRT1 in the regulation of inflammation and metabolic disorders. Cellular Signalling. 2013;**25**:1939-1948. DOI: 10.1016/j.cellsig.2013.06.007

[130] Jäger S, Handschin C, St-Pierre J, Spiegelman BM. AMP-activated protein kinase (AMPK) action in skeletal muscle via direct phosphorylation of PGC-1alpha. Proceedings of the National Academy of Sciences USA. 2007;**104**:12017-12022. DOI: 10.1073/pnas.0705070104

[131] Shaw RJ. LKBI and AMPK control of mTOR signalling and growth. Acta Physiologica. 2009;**196**:65-80. DOI: 10.1111/j.1748-1716.2009.01972.x

[132] Ghosh HS, McBurney M, Robbins PD. SIRT1 negatively regulates the mammalian target of rapamycin. PLoS One. 2010;**5**:e9199. DOI: 10.1371/journal.pone.0009199164

[133] Dan HC, Cooper MJ, Cogswell PC, Duncan JA, Ting JP-Y, Baldwin SAS. Akt-dependent regulation of NF-kB is controlled by mTOR and raptor in association with Ikk. Genes & Development. 2008;**22**:1490-1500. DOI: 10.1101/gad.1662308

[134] Hopkins BD, Goncalves MD, Cantley LC. Insulin-PI3K signalling: An evolutionarily insulated metabolic driver of cancer. Nature Reviews. Endocrinology. 2020;**16**:276-283. DOI: 10.1038/s41574-020-0329-9

[135] Schultze SM, Hemmings BA, NiessenM TO. PI3K/AKT,MAPK and AMPK signalling: Protein kinases in glucose homeostasis. Expert Reviews in Molecular Medicine. 2012;**14**:e1. DOI: 10.1017/S146239941100210

[136] Zhao Y, Hu X, Liu Y, Dong S, Wen Z, He W, et al. ROS signaling under metabolic stress: Crosstalk between AMPK and AKT pathway. Molecular Cancer. 2017;**16**:79. DOI: 10.1186/s12943-017-0648-1

[137] Jiramongkol Y, Lam EW-F. FOXO transcription factor family in cancer and metastasis. Cancer Metastasis Reviews. 2020;**39**:681-709. DOI: 10.1007/s10555-020-09883-w

[138] Zhang X, Tang N, Hadden TJ, Rishi AK. Akt, fox O and regulation of apoptosis. Biochimica et Biophysica Acta. 2011;**1813**:1978-1986. DOI: 10.1016/j.bbamcr.2011.03.010

[139] Wang F, Nguyen M, Qin FX, Tong Q. SIRT2 deacetylates FOXO3a in response to oxidative stress and caloric restriction. Aging Cell. 2007;**6**:505-514. DOI: 10.1111/j.1474-9726.2007.00304.x

[140] Mouchiroud L, Houtkooper RH, Moullan N, Katsyuba E, Ryu D, Canto C, et al. The NAD(+)/Sirtuin pathway modulates longevity through activation of mitochondrial UPR and FOXO signaling. Cell. 2013;**154**:430-441. DOI: 10.1016/j.cell.2013.06.016

[141] Hay N. Interplay between FOXO, TOR, and Akt. Biochimica et Biophysica Acta. 2011;**1813**:1965-1970. DOI: 10.1016/j.bbamcr.2011.03.013

[142] Tzivion G, Dobson M, Ramakrishnan G. Fox O transcription factors; regulation by AKT and 14-3-3 proteins. Biochimica et Biophysica Acta. 2011;**1813**:1938-1945. DOI: 10.1016/j.bbamcr. 2011.06.002

[143] Janku F, Yap TA, Meric-Berstam F. Targeting the PI3K pathway in cancer. Nature Reviews. Clinical Oncology. 2018;**15**:273-291. DOI: 10.1038/nrclinonc.2018.28

[144] Salminen A, Kaarniranta K. AMP-activated protein kinase (AMPK) controls the aging process via an integrated signaling network. Ageing

Research Reviews. 2012;**11**:230-241. DOI: 10.1016/j.arr.2011.12.005

[145] Rutherford C, Speirs C, Williams JJ, Ewart MA, Mancini SJ, Hawley SA, et al. Phosphorylation of Janus kinase 1 (JAK1) by AMP-activated protein kinase (AMPK) links energy sensing to anti-inflammatory signaling. Science Signaling. 2016;**9**(ra109):8566. DOI: 10.1126/scisignal.aaf

Chapter 6

Cardiac Natriuretic Peptide System: A Link between Adipose Tissue, Obesity, and Insulin Resistance

Mustafa Öztop

Abstract

Cardiac natriuretic peptides (NPs) play critical roles in body systems, besides essentially maintaining cardiovascular homeostasis. White adipose tissue exerts functions such as energy storage, hormone secretion, thermal insulation, regulation of insulin sensitization, and prevention of traumatic injuries to vital organs. Brown adipose tissue is a thermogenic tissue that protects the body from cold environments by dissipation of chemical energy derived from fuel substrates as heat. NPs have potent regulatory effects on adipose tissues having high expression of NP receptors. Evidence suggests that the NP system participates in the regulation of adipose tissue metabolism during obesity, insulin resistance, and type 2 diabetes. Reduced NP synthesis and changed clearance receptor expression may adversely affect NPs' target organ metabolism during obesity, insulin resistance, and type 2 diabetes. Defective NP system might lead to adipose tissue dysfunction during obesity, type 2 diabetes, insulin resistance, and cardiovascular disease. Improved NP levels have been associated with positive metabolic outcomes. The positive association between increased NP levels and lower incidence of insulin resistance, obesity, and type 2 diabetes holds promise for future applications of NPs system in clinical settings. This chapter provides an overview of the impact of the NP system on adipose tissue metabolism in cardiometabolic diseases.

Keywords: natriuretic peptide system, adipose tissue, obesity, insulin resistance, type 2 diabetes, thermogenesis

1. Introduction

Natriuretic peptides are hormones that exert cardiovascular and renal effects. Their congenital absence or genetic ablation leads to serious consequences, especially in the cardiovascular system. Thus, cardiovascular health could be improved through genetic and pharmacological manipulation of these natriuretic peptides [1]. Although natriuretic peptides are key players in the regulation of cardiovascular and renal systems, accumulating evidence shows that they could play pivotal roles in counteracting metabolic diseases and conditions such as obesity, type 2 diabetes, and insulin resistance that adversely affect human population across the world. One of the most attractive therapeutic approaches to combat obesity and type 2 diabetes is the activation of brown adipose tissue that has been rediscovered in adult humans in the late 2000s. Stimuli that activate this tissue have been explored in many animal models and in humans [2]. Since the discovery of their potent lipolytic effects on human adipose tissue in the early 2000s [3, 4], many studies have been focused on the effect of natriuretic peptides on glucose and lipid metabolism pathways that are altered in obesity and type 2 diabetes [5]. In addition, promising results came from the studies on activation of brown adipose tissue. These studies reveal that natriuretic peptides might serve as a pathophysiological link between brown adipose tissue activation and metabolic diseases. In fact, obesity, type 2 diabetes, and insulin resistance may commonly manifest in the same patient, all of which are associated with heart failure and development of multiple organ failure due to impaired oxidative metabolism [6]. Therefore, better understanding of the metabolic effects of natriuretic peptides on lipid metabolism during obesity and type 2 diabetes would pave the way for treatment and prevention of those maladies that are blamed for both deaths and impaired quality of life. This chapter provides a general overview of natriuretic peptide system and adipose tissue and discusses genetic, physiological, and pharmacological evidence of natriuretic peptide system linking adipose tissue to obesity and type 2 diabetes.

2. The natriuretic peptide system

2.1 Natriuretic peptides

Natriuretic peptides (NPs) are peptide hormones responsible for maintaining cardiovascular homeostasis. Atrial natriuretic peptide (ANP), brain natriuretic peptide (BNP), and C-type natriuretic peptide (CNP) constitute the main mammalian natriuretic peptide (NP) system [7, 8]. Emerging evidence shows that these peptides play critical roles in different systems of the body [9]. ANP, the first member of the NP system, is mostly produced and stored in the atrial myocytes, and it is released in response to various stimuli such as heart wall stretch and atrial distension [10]. The discovery of ANP led to the assumption that the heart was formerly an endocrine organ. ANP is first generated as a 152-amino-acid precursor, which is subsequently cleaved into its biologically active form by corin, a transmembrane serine protease that works as a pro-atrial natriuretic peptide-converting enzyme [11]. Initially identified in porcine brain, BNP is the second member of the NP system and is also known as a ventricular natriuretic peptide. It is produced as a 134-amino-acid precursor before being processed into its biologically active form [12, 13]. ProBNP-108 and BNP-32 are the two most physiologically active variants of BNP. BNP-32 is mostly expressed in the atria, but proBNP-108 is primarily expressed in the ventricular myocardium. ProBNP-108 is cleaved by furin, a proprotein convertase, to produce BNP-32 and NT (N-Terminal)-BNP-76 [14]. ANP levels rise in response to increased atrial pressures, whereas BNP levels rise in response to ventricular overload [15]. During congestive heart failure and cardiac hypertrophy, both ANP and BNP are substantially expressed by the atrium and ventricle, with BNP expression levels being reported to be excessively higher than ANP levels [16, 17]. Patients affected by hypertension and obesity, on the other hand, were found to have low plasma ANP levels [18] due to reduced natriuretic peptide release and increased natriuretic peptide clearance (depending on natriuretic peptide receptor C overexpression) [19, 20] and/or due to the activation of the renin-angiotensin-aldosterone system [21]. CNP, the third member of the NP system, is derived from a 126-amino-acid precursor, which is subsequently cleaved by furin into two endogenous forms, CNP-53 and CNP-22 [22, 23]. CNP has been found in a variety of organs, including the heart, kidney, lung, endothelial cells, bone, and the central nervous system, despite its low circulating concentration [24, 25]. CNP is primarily involved in vascular homeostasis and has anti-hypertrophic and anti-fibrotic actions on cardiac myocytes and fibroblasts, respectively, due to its endothelial origin [26, 27]. Later on, two new members of the NP system have been discovered. Of those, D-type natriuretic peptide (DNP, also known as Dendroaspis natriuretic peptide) is a physiologically active peptide molecule of 38 amino acids that was first discovered in the venom of the green mamba snake (*Dendroaspis angusticeps*) [28]. Another member of the NP system is urodilatin (URO), which is produced by the distal kidney tubules and is considered as a local part of the natriuretic peptide system due to its diuretic effects. It was first found as a 32-amino-acid peptide in urine [29–31]. Altogether, each endogenous natriuretic peptide is an inseparable component of the cardiovascular system [32]. NPs primarily work on the cardiovascular and renal systems to maintain water-electrolyte balance and blood pressure. The NP system, on the other hand, works to counteract the renin-angiotensin system (RAS) hyperactivity, which results in antimitogenic properties and helps to prevent cardiac hypertrophy and fibrosis. Overall, the NP system stands as a defense mechanism against the damages that hypertension and hypertension-associated diseases might cause [32, 33].

2.2 Natriuretic peptide receptors

The NP signals are conveyed by its transmembrane receptors. A transmembrane natriuretic peptide receptor A (NPRA) is encoded by the *Npr1* gene and has been detected in many tissues including the heart, kidneys, and adipose tissue [34]. NPRA binds ANP and BNP in a selective manner. Upon binding, NPRA is activated through a conformational change in its catalytic domain with intrinsic guanylyl cyclase activity, which consequently results in the conversion of intracellular guanosine triphosphate (GTP) to cyclic guanosine monophosphate (cGMP) [35]. Likewise, natriuretic peptide receptor B (NPRB) encoded by the *Npr2* gene is also a transmembrane receptor [36]. NPRB generates cytoplasmic cGMP from GTP due to intrinsic guanylyl cyclase activity once CNP binds to its extracellular domain [37]. Conversely, *Npr3* gene product, natriuretic peptide receptor C (NPRC), is a transmembrane receptor lacking guanylyl cyclase activity and rather acts as a clearance receptor [38]. NPRC binds all NP ligands (ANP, BNP, and CNP) with similar affinity and sequesters them from the circulation, thereby keeping circulating NP levels within the physiological ranges [39, 40]. In addition to NPRC signaling pathway, ANP and BNP may be cleared from circulation through an alternative pathway catalyzed by neprilysin, a protease that is a membrane-bound zinc-dependent metallopeptidase attacking on amino terminal end of hydrophobic residues [41, 42]. This pathway is of considerable relevance to pathological scenarios such as heart failure that results in increased ANP levels [43]. Given the NP catabolic pathways, the rate of NP clearance from circulation in humans varies depending on the specific type and effects of such peptides [44, 45].

3. Adipose tissue

3.1 Cell type diversity, morphology, and function

Adipose tissue (AT) is a specialized connective tissue that carries out a diverse set of tasks such as energy storage, hormone production, thermal insulation, and thermogenesis [46]. AT, corresponding to roughly 5–50% of human body weight [47], consists of two basic components: cells and extracellular matrix [48]. AT has abundantly adipocytes (also called adipose cells or fat cells), among which other cell types are mesenchymal stem cells, preadipocytes, macrophages, fibroblasts, endothelial cells, and smooth muscle cells [46]. AT is a key player in energy storage and consumption. The excess energy is efficiently stored in the form of neutral triglycerides (TGs) in the AT via lipogenesis, an anabolic pathway encompassing fatty acid synthesis and triglyceride synthesis [49]. On the other hand, when energy consumption is greater than its production, the stored energy is rapidly mobilized to bring into use [50]. This highlights the fact that AT is a dynamically remodelable tissue responsible for storage and reallocation of lipids in response to cellular energy excess or depletion [51]. Furthermore, AT fulfills other physiological tasks and is now regarded as a significant endocrine organ.

AT has been divided into two major subclasses: white adipose tissue (WAT) and brown adipose tissue (BAT). WAT is responsible for the production of some pro-inflammatory cytokines and chemokines, including interleukin 6 (IL-6), IL-18 and tumor necrosis factor-alpha (TNF-α), that modulate inflammation [48, 52]. In addition, adipocytes in WAT (white adipocytes) secrete many adipocyte-derived paracrine and endocrine molecules (collectively called "adipokines"), including leptin and adiponectin that regulate energy metabolism [47, 48]. Leptin is regarded as a master regulator of energy balance. It controls glucose metabolism and energy expenditure and suppresses food intake through binding to the long form of the leptin receptor (LEPR) that is highly expressed in brain areas responsible for the control of feeding and energy expenditure [53]. However, the leptin's ability to lower food consumption is dependent on the melanocortin-3 receptor (MC3R) in the brain, which regulates energy homeostasis [54]. Adiponectin, a well-known homeostatic factor, yields insulin sensitivity-promoting effects by inhibiting hepatic glucose production and stimulating fatty acid oxidation in skeletal muscles [55]. By turning our focus to WAT and BAT below, we give further information about these different types of adipose tissue.

3.2 White adipose tissue

In healthy individuals, WAT makes up at least 10% of the total body weight. Energy storage, hormone secretion, thermal insulation, regulation of insulin sensitivity, and prevention of traumatic injuries to vital organs are among its basic tasks [49]. Adipocytes in the WAT (white adipocytes) have low mitochondrial abundance and store TGs as large intracellular lipid droplets [56]. WAT is mainly subdivided into subcutaneous adipose tissue (SAT) and visceral adipose tissue (VAT) [57]. In humans, SAT is mostly found in the gluteal and femoral regions. It may be divided into two types: deep SAT and superficial SAT, which differ morphologically and metabolically [58]. Deep SAT has been linked to the pathophysiology of obesity-related metabolic complications, whereas superficial SAT is more associated with protective roles against metabolic derangements [59–61]. Located around the internal organs, VAT exists in pericardial, gonadal, omental, mesenteric, and retroperitoneal storages, and protects them from mechanical damage and friction [62]. SAT and VAT show marked differences in adipocyte phenotype, gene expression signature, and lipolytic and endocrine activities [63].

3.3 Brown adipose tissue

BAT, as a thermogenic tissue, protects the body from cold environments by dissipating chemical energy derived from fuel substrates as heat [64]. Brown adipocytes contain many small-sized lipid droplets and copious amounts of mitochondria. They express uncoupling protein 1 (UCP1), also called thermogenin, that uncouples the electron transfer chain from the ATP synthesis to generate heat [65]. Two types of brown adipocytes have been identified. The traditional brown adipocytes are myogenic factor 5-positive (*Myf5+*) cells and are located in the interscapular region in rodents [66]. On the other hand, beige adipocytes are *Myf5*-negative cells interspersed among white adipocytes in the inguinal WAT in rodents. Beige cells are also inducible or recruitable brown adipocytes in WAT [66]. Therefore, beige adipocytes resemble both white adipocytes with regard to their capacity to store energy, and brown adipocytes in terms of their ability to drive thermogenesis [67].

It has long been considered that BAT merely exists in some mammalian species, including human newborns, hibernating animals, and rodents [68–70]. However, recent studies have shown that BAT is metabolically activated in adult humans upon cold exposure [71–73]. Mounting lines of evidence have uncovered the possible mechanisms of action of BAT in counteracting obesity and its coexisting diseases in humans [74]. Some studies have demonstrated that exposure to different cold regimes (e.g., 15–16°C for 6 hours/day for 10 days or 17°C for 2 hours/day for 6 weeks) may stimulate human BAT, enhance non-shivering thermogenesis and reduce body fat mass [75–81]. However, whether these effects might continue in the long-term period (months to years) remain obscure. On the other hand, several studies have revealed that subcutaneously placed embryonic BAT could reverse type 1 diabetes-related parameters in streptozotocin-treated mice, thus improving glucose homeostasis and weight gain and reversing type 1 diabetes independently from insulin [82–85]. The extent to which BAT thermogenesis would influence obesity and diabetes relies on the quantity of actively recruited BAT [62, 86]. Another study reported that some central neural modulators would decrease fat mass and body weight by activating BAT thermogenesis and triggering the switch from white adipocytes to brown adipocytes in order to burn off excess energy [64].

3.4 Adipose tissue as a cardiovascular system modulator

Considering their anatomical localization, cardiac adipose tissue stores can be described as pericardial adipose tissue (PAT) and perivascular adipose tissue (PVAT) [86, 87]. The pericardial adipose tissue consists of paracardial adipose tissue and epicardial adipose tissue (EAT). EAT is a metabolically active tissue, which provides energy supply to myocardium in case of augmented energy demand [88]. Given all the adipose tissue reservoirs, EAT utilizes the lipogenesis and lipolysis pathways at the highest rate. EAT exerts modulatory effects on the vascular tone and coronary artery functions through secretion of molecules such as adipokines and nitric oxide (NO) [86]. EAT has been reported to possess brown/beige adipocyte-specific phenotypes in hibernators and human adults due to its thermogenic capacity [70, 89].

PVAT, which is located around veins, arteries, and small vessels [90], plays an active role in fine-tuning endothelial function, vascular tone, and vascular remodeling, and represents a dual endocrine-paracrine organ that produces various immunomodulatory and vasoactive molecules, in addition to cytokines and adipokines like leptin and adiponectin [91, 92]. PVAT makes up just 0.3% of total adipose tissue mass and can contain various numbers of brown, white, and beige adipocytes based on its location in the body and despite differences in the predominant cell type. Moreover, it has been shown that periaortic adipose tissue at the thoracic region in human adults has beige-like characteristics, whilst coronary PVAT exhibits WAT-like characteristics [90].

3.5 Dysregulation of adipose tissue in obesity and insulin resistance

Obesity is closely related to impaired insulin sensitivity in the liver, skeletal muscles, and white adipose tissue. Obesity-related insulin resistance is one of the most prevalent causes of type 2 diabetes mellitus and is directly linked to diverse cardiometabolic abnormalities including coronary heart disease, atherosclerosis, and hypertension [46, 49, 93]. In response to chronic excessive calorie intake, expansion of adipose tissue through adipocyte hyperplasia (cell number increase) and/or hypertrophy (cell size increase) is a major determinant of metabolic dysfunction and cardiovascular diseases [49, 94]. Hyperplasia might be regarded as a healthy mechanism of AT expansion. However, hypertrophy could lead to adipocyte dysfunction as adipocytes outreach their expansion limits as a result of development of hypoxic conditions, oxidative stress, and pro-inflammatory cytokine release [95]. Thus, the body region where excessive adiposity occurs is one of the most crucial factors identifying the obesity-related cardiometabolic complications [5].

It has been considered that enlargement of VAT has established a strong link between adverse metabolic alterations and increased cardiovascular risk, while expansion of SAT makes a minor contribution to these adverse outcomes [49]. The "portal hypothesis" may account for one of the possible reasons for this difference. The portal hypothesis propounds that visceral fat tissue in obese patients increasingly releases free fatty acids (FFAs) and cytokines into the portal vein, resulting in their accumulation in the liver. Then, hepatic fat accumulation promotes the development of hepatic insulin resistance and type 2 diabetes [96–98]. This condition that increases the amount of FFAs transported to the liver via the portal circulation is also linked to atherogenic lipid profile and hepatic steatosis [98]. Another possible reason for this difference is that VAT is more susceptible to the effects of pro-inflammatory molecules than other adipose tissues, since increased adiposity creates a pro-inflammatory milieu. It has been reported that VAT has higher expression and secretion of several pro-inflammatory mediators including TNF-α and IL-6, as compared to SAT [99, 100]. Augmented expression of pro-inflammatory cytokines causes phosphorylation of serine/threonine residues of insulin receptor substrate proteins, leading to dissociation of insulin receptor substrate proteins from effector proteins in the insulin signaling cascade pathway and resulting in the development of insulin resistance [101]. In addition, pro-inflammatory cytokines cause local and systemic inflammation by triggering recruitment of macrophages and T-lymphocytes to the relevant sites [102]. Resident macrophages play a crucial role in the promotion and perpetuation of adipocyte dysregulation and insulin resistance. Furthermore, experimental evidence shows that necrotic cell death in adipose tissue over the course of obesity might induce the recruitment of pro-inflammatory M1 macrophages, which produce multiple pro-inflammatory cytokines that exacerbate chronic inflammation and insulin resistance [103]. Additionally, it has been shown that anti-inflammatory adiponectin is expressed at a lower level in VAT than in SAT and its circulating concentrations are reduced in obese people with augmented visceral fat accumulation [104].

SAT has a restricted potential to expand owing to its poor adipogenesis capability. This limited capacity results in adipocyte hypertrophy, promoting the formation of fat storages in non-adipose tissues such as in the heart, liver, and skeletal muscles [105]. This deleterious mechanism of adipogenesis is also regarded as "lipotoxicity" and is linked to the development of systemic insulin resistance and enhanced risk of type 2 diabetes. It has been put forward that intrahepatic content of TGs represents a more acceptable marker of insulin resistance than VAT [106]. On the other hand, PVAT exhibits hyperplastic and hypertrophic characteristics in obesity [107]. It has been propounded that "obesity triad" encompassing oxidative stress, inflammation, and hypoxia might be the major mechanism responsible for PVAT dysfunction in obesity. Adipocyte dysfunction during obesity arises from the "whitening" of PVAT, which creates a hypoxic and pro-inflammatory milieu affecting the vasculature [86]. Moreover, reduced adiponectin production by PVAT in obesity promotes endothelial dysfunction [108]. In this respect, studies using genetically-modified and diet-induced animal models of obesity revealed that anticontractile properties of PVAT are totally lost [49].

Adequate insulin signaling in AT is a crucial factor in the maintenance of systemic blood glucose homeostasis, as evidenced by a number of mice models, even though skeletal muscle is responsible for the bulk of insulin-stimulated glucose uptake [109]. Adipocyte-specific glucose transporter type 4 (GLUT4) knockout in mice affects skeletal muscle and liver insulin signaling, which results in glucose intolerance, insulin resistance, and hyperinsulinemia [110]. Adipocyte-specific insulin receptor-knockout mice exhibited basal glucose uptake in a similar fashion, but insulin-stimulated glucose uptake by adipocytes was considerably lower than in controls. These mice had improved systemic glucose tolerance [111]. It is worthy to note that this difference might arise from the activation of alternative signaling pathways to compensate for the innate lack of adipocyte insulin signaling pathway. A recent study on adipocyte-specific insulin receptor (IR) and insulin-like growth factor 1 receptor (IGF-1R) knockout (one of these receptors: IRKO, IGF-1RKO or both of them: double KO, DKO) mice found that while all KO groups had equivalent or lower fat mass than controls, IRKO and DKO mice showed systemic insulin resistance and hepatic steatosis in comparison with the controls and IGF-1RKO groups. The combined ablation of these receptors led to serious glucose homeostasis disturbances [112]. Together, these findings indicate that when there are deficiencies in insulin receptor signaling in the innate AT, a compensatory mechanism may be triggered possibly through insulin-independent signaling pathways in other insulin-responsive tissues in order to counteract systemic glucose intolerance. However, this evidence suggests that adequate insulin signaling inside the AT is critical for overall health.

Impacts of AT insulin sensitivity on systemic health may be mediated by the regulation of adipose tissue lipolysis that breaks down triglycerides into FFAs and glycerol. Situations like fasting, exercise, and stress induce lipolysis through adrenergic activation, thus mobilizing energy storage. In case of fed state, insulin inhibits lipolysis in the direction of lipid storage. As a result, defective insulin signaling in AT could lead to an increase in basal lipolysis rate [113]. Since the inflammatory cytokine TNF may stimulate lipolysis independently of insulin signaling, chronic low-grade inflammation caused by obesity may also trigger excessive FFA release by adipocytes and promote lipotoxicity and lipid-induced insulin resistance [114, 115]. Obesity and insulin resistance have extensively been linked to elevated rates of basal lipolysis. The ensuing rise in circulating FFA levels increases metabolic dysfunction by promoting lipid accumulation in the liver and muscle [113]. Disturbances in lipid storage, such as those caused by obesity or lipodystrophy, can impair adipocyte function and lead to insulin resistance. Insulin resistance in the adipose tissue disrupts normal adipocyte signaling and metabolism, leading to an increase in lipolysis. Ectopic lipid accumulation and insulin resistance in other tissues, such as skeletal muscle and liver, can result from chronically increased circulating lipids. Insulin resistance in the liver is deleterious because insulin signaling controls hepatic glucose synthesis. All of these events have the potential to produce a major effect on metabolic health, culminating in a vicious cycle that perpetuates systemic metabolic illness [48, 113]. Type 2 diabetes and hepatic lipid accumulation are common in situations with high basal lipolysis, such as Cushing's syndrome [116, 117], as well as in cases of lipoatrophy when circulating lipids are excessive [118]. Although the bulk of whole-body glucose uptake could not have been directly taken up by AT, it is obvious that impairment in glucose uptake and lipid accumulation in AT have an impact on other insulin-responsive organs, modulating the overall status of systemic health [48]. Much more remains to be found out how altered adipose tissue metabolism is going to contribute to metabolic conditions such as obesity, insulin resistance, and type 2 diabetes.

4. Natriuretic peptides as key players in adipose tissue dysfunction, obesity, and insulin resistance

4.1 Physiological actions of natriuretic peptides on adipose tissue

Currently, NPs have been well established to be powerful metabolic hormones that are responsible for the fulfillment of key functions in adipose tissue having high expression of NP receptors [119]. Demonstration of ANP mRNA expression by human adipose tissue is a strong indication that ANP exerts autocrine/paracrine effects on this tissue [120]. In 2000, it was evidenced that, in the potency order of ANP > BNP> > CNP, NPs exert potent lipolytic effects on human adipose tissue in both *in vivo* and *in vitro* circumstances [3]. This seminal observation has unveiled a novel pathway orchestrating human adipose tissue lipolysis in a cGMP-dependent manner, that does not require phosphodiesterase 3B (PDE3B) inhibition and cyclic adenosine monophosphate (cAMP) production [3]. While ANP exerts its lipolytic effects through binding to its receptor NPRA with augmented cGMP production and lipase activation [3], CNP produces its lipolytic effects on human preadipocytes by binding to its receptor NPRB and triggering cGMP synthesis [121]. In addition, increased mRNA levels of genes involved in adipogenesis have shown that CNP might govern the process of adipogenesis [121]. Furthermore, a recent study has reported that endothelial overexpression of CNP in transgenic mice (in which CNP was placed under the control of the Tie2 promoter) suppresses adipocyte hypertrophy and lipogenesis in WAT while stimulating BAT thermogenesis and increasing energy expenditure [122]. On the other hand, expression of NPRC in human adipocytes is essential to the effectiveness of the NP system in adipose tissue. It has been hypothesized that the metabolic effects of NPs may depend on the relative tissue ratio of NPRA to NPRC, which has functional importance for physiological actions of NPs [123, 124]. An *in vivo* and *in vitro* study corroborating this hypothesis showed that rodent adipocytes with a considerably higher ratio of NPRC to NPRA did not respond to lipolytic effects of endogenous and exogenous ANP [4].

NPs play additional roles in modulating the release of adipokines and cytokines from adipose tissue. When ANP is added to isolated human adipocytes *in vitro*, it inhibits leptin secretion [125]. An *in vitro* study found that ANP and BNP augmented adiponectin mRNA expression and production in human adipocytes, a modulatory effect that is inhibited by preincubation with HS142-1 acting as a selective NPRA antagonist [126]. ANP generated an inhibitory effect on production of pro-inflammatory cytokines such as TNF-α and IL-6 from macrophages and adipocytes [24]. Taken all together, these effects show that situations of low-grade inflammation in adipose tissue during obesity and insulin resistance would have been positively affected by activation of NPRA. It has been reported that NPs could stimulate the thermogenic program of brown adipocytes from BAT. NPRA activated by ANP triggers cGMP rise and protein kinase G (PKG) activation. PKG then activates p38 mitogen-activated protein kinase (p38-MAPK). In mouse and human adipocytes, this activation cascade leads to increased mitochondrial biogenesis and to activation of key thermogenic protein UCP1 and gene expression programs responsible for fatty acid oxidation [124, 127]. When exposed to cold conditions, mice exhibited a rise in NPRA expression and circulating NPs concentrations but a decline in NPRC expression in WAT and BAT, suggesting an increase in NPs-induced formation of beige adipocytes [128]. On the contrary, inactivation of ANP gene in mice led to an impairment in triglyceride and glycogen metabolism in the liver and to a decline in cold tolerance and BAT thermogenesis [129]. Browning of WAT was observed in NPRC knockout mice ($NPRC^{-}/^{-}$) [127]. Based on all these results, we may strongly support the assertion that NPs are crucial in promoting the conversion of white to brown adipocytes to increase energy expenditure and reduce the white fat mass.

The relevant clinical implications of administering NPs as metabolic hormones have been excellently reviewed [22]. Intravenous infusion of ANP in lean and obese human subjects led to a remarkable rise in plasma FFA and glycerol concentrations, indicating lipid mobilization. Microdialysis data in subcutaneous abdominal adipose tissue also revealed that both groups had an increase in the extracellular glycerol concentration during ANP administration [130, 131]. However, this increase was not reversed with the use of propranolol, a β-adrenergic receptor antagonist used to blunt β-adrenergic effect of catecholamines on adipose tissue [130]. This finding supports the fact that ANP is a powerful lipolytic hormone that acts independently of the activation of the sympathetic nervous system [130, 131]. It is generally known that, during exercise, the heart releases ANP and BNP into the bloodstream [132]. The increment in ANP and BNP levels in the bloodstream during exercise is a robust indicator of contribution to enhanced energy supply [123]. Similarly, plasma adiponectin concentrations increased in both healthy volunteers [133] and patients with heart failure [126, 134] after intravenous injection of human ANP.

4.2 Dysregulation of natriuretic peptide system in obesity and insulin resistance

Considering the link between NPs and their receptors, cardiometabolic diseases, insulin resistance, type 2 diabetes, and obesity, substantial progress has been made in the knowledge of metabolic effects of NPs during recent decades (**Figure 1**). For example, NPs are implicated in many processes including improvement in insulin resistance and induction of lipolysis. Multiple lines of evidence suggest that NPs act as key players in the regulation of metabolic pathways and in the pathophysiology

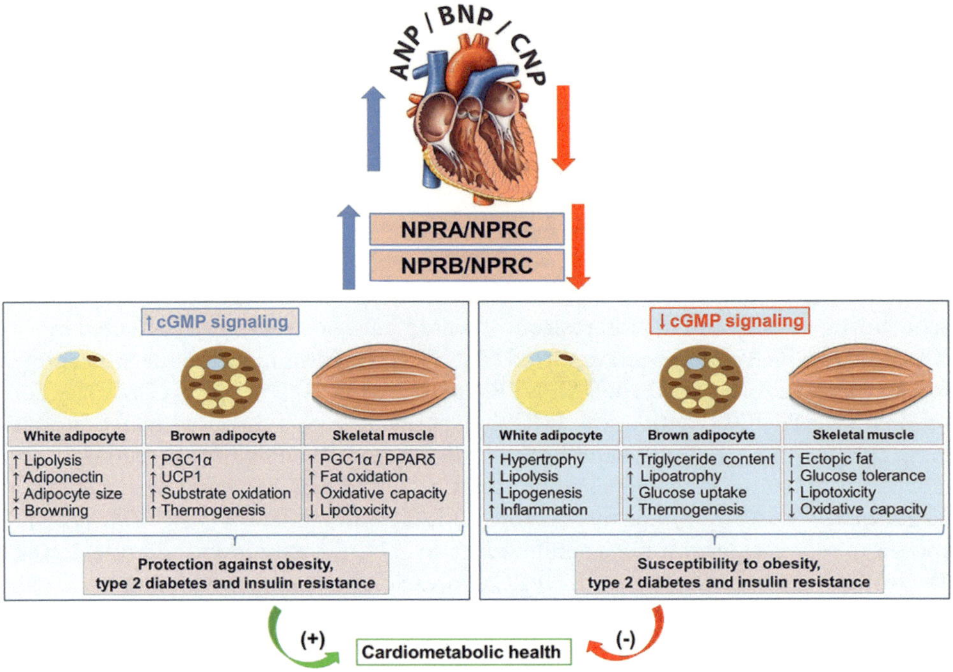

Figure 1.
Involvement of natriuretic peptides and their receptors in the pathophysiology of obesity, type 2 diabetes, and insulin resistance, with possible implications for cardiometabolic health. Natriuretic peptide signaling evoked through the NPRA and NPRB starts with cGMP signaling, which enhances lipolysis in white adipose tissue, thermogenesis in brown adipose tissue, and oxidative capacity in skeletal muscle under physiological circumstances. These physiological actions protect against obesity, type 2 diabetes, and insulin resistance, thus providing significant cardiometabolic health benefits. In pathological settings, changes in the NPRA/NPRC and NPRB/NPRC ratios in favor of NPRC result in reduced natriuretic peptide production and release, and in increased clearance receptor function. Obesity, type 2 diabetes, and related comorbidities compromise cardiometabolic health and are all partly consequences of the aforementioned alterations in the natriuretic peptide system. ANP, atrial natriuretic peptide; BNP, brain natriuretic peptide; cGMP, cyclic guanosine monophosphate; CNP, C-type natriuretic peptide; NPRA, natriuretic peptide receptor A; NPRB, natriuretic peptide receptor B; NPRC, natriuretic peptide receptor C; PGC1α, peroxisome proliferator-activated receptor-gamma coactivator 1-alpha; PPARδ, peroxisome proliferator-activated receptor-delta; UCP1, uncoupling protein 1.

of cardiometabolic diseases, obesity, and type 2 diabetes [22]. The lower availability of NPs could be attributable to their decreased production and release as well as to the increased function of their clearance receptor. Animal experiments revealed that diabetic obese db/db mice and obese Zucker fatty rats have lower cardiac ANP and BNP expression at the mRNA level [135, 136]. However, feeding mice with a high-fat diet had no effect on their plasma BNP levels [137]. NPRC mRNA level rose in the heart of db/db mice [125], but NPRA and NPRC expression decreased and increased, respectively, in white and brown adipose tissue of db/db mice [137]. Moreover, obese mice fed a high-fat diet had increased levels of endopeptidase and neprilysin (which are responsible for NP breakdown) in plasma and in mesenteric fat, indicating a higher NP clearance [138].

Insulin resistance, type 2 diabetes, and obesity have all been reported to be inversely associated with human plasma NPs [6]. Obese people showed lower plasma BNP levels than non-obese people, indicating a negative relationship between body mass index (BMI) and BNP levels [139]. A cohort study revealed that plasma NT-proANP and NT-proBNP concentrations were inversely related to obesity and to all other components of the metabolic syndrome, with the exception of hypertension [140]. VAT and hepatic fat mass in patients with heart failure were found to be adversely associated with BNP and NT-proBNP plasma levels. In addition, a link between reduced circulating NP levels and altered AT distribution was also found. Elevated levels of NPs, on the other hand, have been reported to be a stronger indicator of obesity profile [141]. The NPRA to NPRC ratio decreased in the adipose tissue of obese patients with type 2 diabetes, indicating increased NP clearance. Treatment with pioglitazone increased the NPRA to NPRC ratio as well as the insulin sensitivity, indicating that a lower NPRA to NPRC ratio is linked to glucose intolerance and insulin resistance [142]. Obese patients also exhibited high neprilysin expression, indicating that NPs break down rapidly and their effects lessen [138]. Overall, these findings suggest that reduced circulating NP levels are closely associated with the progression of numerous metabolic disorders, including type 2 diabetes and obesity. Currently, the capacity of neprilysin inhibitors, such as sacubitril, to raise NP levels is being considered as one of the major strategies for improving the metabolic profile in type 2 diabetes and obesity through remodeling adipose tissue [143]. Nevertheless, further research and clinical trials are required to obtain the optimal metabolic benefits from those drugs and to maximize their effects.

The relevance of NP receptors and signaling cascade components in metabolic function research has been demonstrated using genetically engineered mouse models. Body weight and fat mass were reduced in NPRC knockout mice ($NPRC^{-}/^{-}$). Furthermore, adding ANP to adipocyte culture from NPRC knockout mice boosted UCP1 expression, resulting in lipolysis [127]. In comparison to wild-type counterparts, adipocyte-specific NPRC knockout mice ($Nprc^{AKO}$) showed higher thermogenesis, improved insulin sensitivity, and increased glucose uptake into BAT. This recent finding also indicated that NPRC knockout mice were protected from developing insulin resistance and obesity as a result of a high-fat diet. Furthermore, in this diet-induced model of insulin resistance and obesity, adipocyte-specific NPRC deletion inhibited the development of inflammation [144]. The knockout of the NPRA gene, however, has been linked to increased fat mass and cardiac hypertrophy [145]. Guanylyl cyclase-A (GCA) heterozygous knockout [GCA(+/−)] mice fed a high-fat diet gained weight and developed glucose intolerance [144, 146]. However, mice overexpressing PKG (cGK-Tg mice) fed a high-fat diet had lower body weight, less visceral and subcutaneous fat depots, and less ectopic fat deposition, thereby showing a significant enhancement in insulin sensitivity and glucose tolerance [146]. Overall, these data suggest that the NPs/guanylyl cyclase (GC) cascades play a crucial role in conferring resistance to obesity and glucose intolerance. Besides, mice overexpressing BNP (BNP-Tg mice) fed a high-fat diet, had better body weight, and glucose tolerance, indicating that BNP attenuates diet-related obesity and insulin resistance [146]. A recent study conducted on mice overexpressing CNP, specifically in adipocytes (A-CNP-Tg mice), showed better glucose tolerance and insulin sensitivity in another model of high-fat diet-induced obesity, which was linked to increased insulin-stimulated protein kinase B (Akt) phosphorylation. These findings imply that adipocyte-specific CNP overexpression offers protection against adipocyte hypertrophy, increased lipid metabolism, inflammation, and impaired insulin sensitivity during high-fat diet-induced obesity [147].

Insulin resistance, increased lipotoxicity, and reduced-fat oxidative capacity are all linked to faulty NPR signaling in skeletal muscle during obesity. The physiologic activation of NPRA by circulating NP is further inhibited by upregulation of NPRC in skeletal muscle as glucose tolerance impairs with obesity [137]. In humans, a substantial positive relationship was initially discovered between insulin sensitivity and muscle NPRA protein expression, as evaluated by hyperinsulinemic-euglycemic clamp at a dosage that primarily shows insulin sensitivity in skeletal muscle [137]. However, the finding of a negative relationship between body fat and muscle NPRA expression is in line with the negative relationship between total saturated ceramide concentration and muscle NPRA expression, two parameters that adversely influence skeletal muscle and whole-body insulin sensitivity [137, 148, 149]. Coué et al. first documented a functional link between insulin sensitivity and skeletal muscle NPRA signaling, indicating that NPR signaling in skeletal muscle may alter insulin sensitivity in addition to plasma NP levels [137]. Furthermore, muscle NPRA protein was significantly reduced in obese people, but it increased in response to diet-induced weight loss and improved insulin sensitivity. Although the molecular mechanisms that modulate muscle NPRA protein expression remain elusive, the aforementioned findings suggest that muscle NPRA acts as a major determinant of insulin sensitivity [137]. Furthermore, as glucose tolerance deteriorates in obese with impaired glucose tolerance (IGT) and type 2 diabetes, overexpression of muscle NPRC might further suppress the physiologic activation of muscle NPRA, which ultimately results in NP system dysfunction. Given that muscle mass accounts for up to 40% of total body weight, even a small increase in muscle NPRC expression could significantly reduce plasma NP levels by increasing NP clearance rates [137, 150]. As glucose tolerance deteriorates independently of blood glucose concentrations in obese patients, muscle NPRC may be activated by high blood insulin levels, as it has previously been established in adipose tissue [150]. Despite the fact that the obese controls and IGT/type 2 diabetes groups were not age-matched, enhanced NPRC expression in skeletal muscle appeared to be independent of age, since there was no relationship between age and muscle NPRC protein expression [137]. These findings in human muscle were mainly duplicated in obese diabetic mice. Obese diabetic mice had higher levels of NPRC protein in their skeletal muscle, white fat, and brown fat, but only muscle NPRC protein was negatively correlated with plasma BNP levels, suggesting that increased plasma BNP clearance by the muscle could contribute to the NP system dysfunction seen in these mice. Findings by Birkenfeld et al. [133] are consistent with previous studies that have linked higher NPRC mRNA levels in white fat to metabolic impairment in rats and humans [146, 151, 152]. These results have also provided a molecular explanation for the close relationship between NP system dysfunction and insulin resistance in humans, irrespective of adiposity [153]. The concept of NP system dysfunction is corroborated by the results reporting that in NPRC knockout mice blood circulation half-life of NPs and their biological activity in target tissues is dramatically enhanced [154]. More importantly, altered NPRA-to-NPRC protein ratio in skeletal muscle was followed by a significant change in p38 MAPK phosphorylation in db/db versus db/+ animals, indicating a possible signaling impairment, given that p38 MAPK is a typical downstream molecular effector of the NPR signaling pathway [127]. Another study has recently reported that protection against diet-induced obesity and insulin resistance had been attributed to NPRC deletion in adipose tissue ($Nprc^{AKO}$) but not in skeletal muscle ($Nprc^{MKO}$). $Nprc^{AKO}$ mice had less inflammation and enhanced energy expenditure, shifting lipid storage from liver to visceral fat. These data led to the conclusion that, when fed a high-fat diet, mouse adipose tissue devoid of NPRC is the primary location of NP-driven metabolic changes [144].

5. Conclusion

Evidence is accumulating that NPs participate in the physiological and pathophysiological regulation of many metabolic diseases including obesity, insulin resistance, and type 2 diabetes, in addition to their well-known actions in the cardiac, vascular, and renal systems. Although there are some conflicting results of the relationship between NP system deficiency and metabolic diseases, many recent studies have shown that the NP system is defective in those diseases. Reduced NPs synthesis, increased clearance, and/or altered NP receptor expression may impair the positive effects of NPs on target metabolic organs such as heart, skeletal muscle, and adipose tissue during obesity, insulin resistance, and type 2 diabetes. Impaired NPs system signaling causes lipid accumulation in adipose tissue, which leads to visceral adiposity, obesity, insulin resistance, type 2 diabetes, and cardiovascular disease. The strong links between adipose tissue enlargement and dysfunction during obesity, insulin resistance, type 2 diabetes, and cardiovascular disease may have been explained by a number of metabolic pathways that are interrelated in the heart, liver, and skeletal muscles. In this perspective, NP insufficiency might be considered one of the pathways linking adipose tissue dysfunction to obesity, type 2 diabetes, insulin resistance, and cardiovascular disease. There is ample data showing that restoring NPs levels after NP injection leads to positive metabolic outcomes, which supports this idea. The positive association between increased levels of NPs and lower incidence of insulin resistance, obesity, and type 2 diabetes holds promise for future NPs applications. Adipocyte hypertrophy, increased lipid synthesis, and visceral and ectopic fat deposition are all prevented by NPs. Furthermore, promising approaches to converting white adipose tissue into thermogenic brown adipose tissue could offer an effective tool for correcting dysfunctional lipid metabolism during obesity, insulin resistance, type 2 diabetes, and cardiovascular disease. In addition, translation of these promising results into clinical practice would open new avenues to treat obesity, type 2 diabetes, and associated diseases. Therefore, further research is needed to completely comprehend the complex interplay between NP system and adipose tissue, heart, liver and skeletal muscles during obesity, insulin resistance, and type 2 diabetes.

Conflict of interest

The author declares no conflict of interest.

Author details

Mustafa Öztop
Faculty of Science and Art, Department of Biology, Burdur Mehmet Akif Ersoy University, Burdur, Turkey

*Address all correspondence to: mustafamalatya@gmail.com

References

[1] Holditch SJ, Schreiber CA, Nini R, Tonne JM, Peng KW, Geurts A, et al. B-type natriuretic peptide deletion leads to progressive hypertension, associated organ damage, and reduced survival: Novel model for human hypertension. Hypertension. 2015;**66**:199-210. DOI: 10.1161/HYPERTENSIONAHA.115.05610

[2] Lapa C, Arias-Loza P, Hayakawa N, Wakabayashi H, Werner RA, Chen X, et al. Whitening and impaired glucose utilization of brown adipose tissue in a rat model of type 2 diabetes mellitus. Scientific Reports. 2017;**7**(1):16795. DOI: 10.1038/s41598-017-17148-w

[3] Sengenès C, Berlan M, De Glisezinski I, Lafontan M, Galitzky J. Natriuretic peptides: A new lipolytic pathway in human adipocytes. The FASEB Journal. 2000;**14**(10):1345-1351. DOI: 10.1096/fasebj.14.10.1345

[4] Sengenès C, Zakaroff-Girard A, Moulin A, Berlan M, Bouloumié A, et al. Natriuretic peptide-dependent lipolysis in fat cells is a primate specificity. American Journal of Physiology. Regulatory, Integrative and Comparative Physiology. 2002;**283**(1):R257-R265. DOI: 10.1152/ajpregu.00453.2001

[5] Rukavina Mikusic NL, Kouyoumdzian NM, Puyó AM, Fernández BE, Choi MR. Role of natriuretic peptides in the cardiovascular-adipose communication: A tale of two organs. Pflügers Archives. 2022;**474**(1):5-19. DOI: 10.1007/s00424-021-02596-1

[6] Jordan J, Birkenfeld AL, Melander O, Moro C. Natriuretic peptides in cardiovascular and metabolic crosstalk: Implications for hypertension management. Hypertension. 2018;**72**(2):270-276. DOI: 10.1161/HYPERTENSIONAHA.118.11081

[7] Woodard GE, Rosado JA. Natriuretic peptides in vascular physiology and pathology. International Review of Cell and Molecular Biology. 2008;**268**:59-93. DOI: 10.1016/S1937-6448(08)00803-4

[8] Pandey K. Emerging roles of natriuretic peptides and their receptors in pathophysiology of hypertension and cardiovascular regulation. Journal of the American Society of Hypertension. 2008;**2**:210-226. DOI: 10.1016/j.jash.2008.02.001

[9] Potter LR, Yoder AR, Flora DR, Antos LK, Dickey DM. Natriuretic peptides: Their structures, receptors, physiologic functions and therapeutic applications. Handbook of Experimental Pharmacology. 2009;**191**:341-366. DOI: 10.1007/978-3-540-68964-5_15

[10] Chun YS, Hyun JY, Kwak YG, Kim IS, Kim CH, et al. Hypoxic activation of the atrial natriuretic peptide gene promoter through direct and indirect actions of hypoxia-inducible factor-1. The Biochemical Journal. 2003;**370**(Pt 1):149-157. DOI: 10.1042/BJ20021087

[11] Yan W, Wu F, Morser J, Wu Q. Corin, a transmembrane cardiac serine protease, acts as a pro-atrial natriuretic peptide-converting enzyme. Proceedings of the National Academy of Science USA. 2000;**97**(15):8525-8529. DOI: 10.1073/pnas.150149097

[12] Hayek S, Nemer M. Cardiac natriuretic peptides: From basic discovery to clinical practice. Cardiovascular Therapeutics. 2011;**29**(6):362-376. DOI: 10.1111/j.1755-5922.2010.00152.x

[13] Sudoh T, Kangawa K, Minamino N, Matsuo H. A new natriuretic peptide in porcine brain. Nature. 1998;**332**(6159): 78-81. DOI: 10.1038/332078a0

[14] Nishikimi T, Minamino N, Ikeda M, Takeda Y, Tadokoro K, et al. Diversity of molecular forms of plasma brain natriuretic peptide in heart failure—Different proBNP-108 to BNP-32 ratios in atrial and ventricular overload. Heart. 2010;**96**(6):432-439. DOI: 10.1136/hrt.2009.178392

[15] Nishikimi T, Kuwahara K, Nakao K. Current biochemistry, molecular biology, and clinical relevance of natriuretic peptides. Journal of Cardiology. 2011;**57**(2):131-140. DOI: 10.1016/j.jjcc.2011.01.002

[16] Mukoyama M, Nakao K, Hosoda K, Suga S, Saito Y, et al. Brain natriuretic peptide as a novel cardiac hormone in humans. Evidence for an exquisite dual natriuretic peptide system, atrial natriuretic peptide and brain natriuretic peptide. The Journal of Clinical Investigation. 1991;**87**(4):1402-1412. DOI: 10.1172/JCI115146

[17] Nakagawa Y, Nishikimi T, Kuwahara K. Atrial and brain natriuretic peptides: Hormones secreted from the heart. Peptides. 2019;**111**:18-25. DOI: 10.1016/j.peptides.2018.05.012

[18] Asferg CL, Nielsen SJ, Andersen UB, Linneberg A, Moller DV, et al. Relative atrial natriuretic peptide deficiency and inadequate renin and angiotensin II suppression in obese hypertensive men. Hypertension. 2013;**62**(1):147-153

[19] Dessì-Fulgheri P, Sarzani R, Tamburrini P, Moraca A, Espinosa E, Cola G, et al. Plasma atrial natriuretic peptide and natriuretic peptide receptor gene expression in adipose tissue of normotensive and hypertensive obese patients. Journal of Hypertension. 1997;**15**(12 Pt 2):1695-1699. DOI: 10.1097/00004872-199715120-00074

[20] Haufe S, Kaminski J, Utz W, Haas V, Mähler A, Daniels MA, et al. Differential response of the natriuretic peptide system to weight loss and exercise in overweight or obese patients. Journal of Hypertension. 2015;**33**(7):1458-1464. DOI: 10.1097/HJH.0000000000000573

[21] Thethi T, Kamiyama M, Kobori H. The link between the renin-angiotensin-aldosterone system and renal injury in obesity and the metabolic syndrome. Current Hypertension Reports. 2012;**14**(2):160-169. DOI: 10.1007/s11906-012-0245-z

[22] Vinnakota S, Chen HH. The importance of natriuretic peptides in cardiometabolic diseases. Journal of Endocrinology. 2020;**4**(6):bvaa052

[23] Wu C, Wu F, Pan J, Morser J, Wu Q. Furin-mediated processing of Pro-C-type natriuretic peptide. The Journal of Biological Chemistry. 2003;**278**(28):25847-25852. DOI: 10.1074/jbc.M301223200

[24] Moro C, Klimcakova E, Lolmède K, Berlan M, Lafontan M, et al. Atrial natriuretic peptide inhibits the production of adipokines and cytokines linked to inflammation and insulin resistance in human subcutaneous adipose tissue. Diabetologia. 2007;**50**(5):1038-1047. DOI: 10.1007/s00125-007-0614-3

[25] Moyes AJ, Hobbs AJ. C-type natriuretic peptide: A multifaceted paracrine regulator in the heart and vasculature. International Journal of Molecular Sciences. 2019;**20**(9):2281. DOI: 10.3390/ijms20092281

[26] Matsuo A, Nagai-Okatani C, Nishigori M, Kangawa K, Minamino N. Natriuretic peptides in human heart: Novel insight into their molecular forms, functions, and diagnostic use. Peptides. 2019;**111**:3-17. DOI: 10.1016/j.peptides.2018.08.006

[27] Villar IC, Panayiotou CM, Sheraz A, Madhani M, Scotland RS, et al. Definitive role for natriuretic peptide receptor-C in mediating the vasorelaxant activity of C-type natriuretic peptide and endothelium-derived hyperpolarizing factor. Cardiovascular Research. 2007;**74**(3):515-525. DOI: 10.1016/j.cardiores.2007.02.032

[28] Schweitz H, Vigne P, Moinier D, Frelin CH, Lazdunski M. A new member of the natriuretic peptide family is present in the venom of the green mamba (*Dendroaspis angusticeps*). The Journal of Biological Chemistry. 1992;**267**(20):13928-13932. DOI: 10.1016/S0021-9258(19)49658-0

[29] Choi MR, Citarella MR, Lee BM, Lucano F, Fernández BE. Urodilatin increases renal dopamine uptake: Intracellular network involved. Journal of Physiology and Biochemistry. 2011;**67**(2):243-247. DOI: 10.1007/s13105-010-0069-8

[30] Citarella MR, Choi MR, Gironacci MM, Medici C, Correa AH, et al. Urodilatin and dopamine: A new interaction in the kidney. Regulatory Peptides. 2009;**153**(1-3):19-24. DOI: 10.1016/j.regpep.2008.11.009

[31] Schulz-Knappe P, Forssmann K, Herbst F, Hock D, Pipkorn R, et al. Isolation and structural analysis of "urodilatin", a new peptide of the cardiodilatin-(ANP)-family, extracted from human urine. Klinische Wochenschrift. 1998;**66**(17):752-759. DOI: 10.1007/BF01726570

[32] Rubattu S, Forte M, Marchitti S, Volpe M. Molecular implications of natriuretic peptides in the protection from hypertension and target organ damage development. International Journal of Molecular Sciences. 2019;**20**(4):798. DOI: 10.3390/ijms20040798

[33] Pandey KN. Molecular and genetic aspects of guanylyl cyclase natriuretic peptide receptor-A in regulation of blood pressure and renal function. Physiological Genomics. 2018;**50**(11):913-928. DOI: 10.1152/physiolgenomics.00083.2018

[34] Rukavina Mikusic NL, Rosón MI, Kouyoumdzian NM, Cantú SM, Fernández BE, et al. Natriuretic peptide receptor type A (NPRA). In: Choi S, editor. Encyclopedia of Signaling Molecules. 2nd ed. New York: Springer; 2018. pp. 3344-3351. DOI: 10.1007/978-3-319-67199-4_101545

[35] Pandey KN, Singh S. Molecular cloning and expression of murine guanylate cyclase/atrial natriuretic factor receptor cDNA. The Journal of Biological Chemistry. 1990;**265**(21):12342-12348. DOI: 10.1016/S0021-9258(19)38352-8

[36] Schulz S. C-type natriuretic peptide and guanylyl cyclase B receptor. Peptides. 2005;**26**:1024-1034. DOI: 10.1016/j.peptides.2004.08.027

[37] Lincoln TM, Cornwell TL. Intracellular cyclic GMP receptor proteins. The FASEB Journal. 1993;7:328-338. DOI: 10.1096/fasebj.7.2.7680013

[38] Jaubert J, Jaubert F, Martin N, Washburn LL, Lee BK, Eicher EM, et al. Three new allelic mouse mutations that cause skeletal overgrowth involve the natriuretic peptide receptor C gene (Npr3). Proceedings of the National Academy of Science USA.

1999;**96**(18):10278-10283. DOI: 10.1073/pnas.96.18.10278

[39] Fuller F, Porter JG, Arfsten AE, Miller J, Schilling JW, et al. Atrial natriuretic peptide clearance receptor. Complete sequence and functional expression of cDNA clones. The Journal of Biological Chemistry. 1988;**263**(19):9395-9401. DOI: 10.1016/S0021-9258(19)76554-5

[40] Zhao J, Pei L. Cardiac endocrinology: Heart-derived hormones in physiology and disease. JACC Basic Translational Science. 2020;**5**(9):949-960. DOI: 10.1016/j.jacbts.2020.05.007

[41] Yandle TG, Brennan SO, Espiner EA, Nicholls MG, Richards AM. Endopeptidase-24.11 in human plasma degrades atrial natriuretic factor (ANF) to ANF(99-105/106-126). Peptides. 1989;**10**(4):891-894. DOI: 10.1016/0196-9781(89)90131-9

[42] Pankow K, Wang Y, Gembardt F, Krause E, Sun X, et al. Successive action of meprin A and neprilysin catabolizes B-type natriuretic peptide. Circulation Research. 2007;**101**(9):875-882. DOI: 10.1161/CIRCRESAHA.107.153585

[43] Potter LR. Natriuretic peptide metabolism, clearance and degradation. The FEBS Journal. 2011;**278**(11):1808-1817. DOI: 10.1111/j.1742-4658.2011.08082.x

[44] Holmes SJ, Espiner EA, Richards AM, Yandle TG, Frampton C. Renal, endocrine, and hemodynamic effects of human brain natriuretic peptide in normal man. The Journal of Clinical Endocrinology and Metabolism. 1993;**76**(1):91-96. DOI: 10.1210/jcem.76.1.8380606

[45] Hunt PJ, Richards AM, Espiner EA, Nicholls MG, Yandle TG. Bioactivity and metabolism of C-type natriuretic peptide in normal man. The Journal of Clinical Endocrinology and Metabolism. 1994;**78**(6):1428-1435. DOI: 10.1210/jcem.78.6.8200946

[46] Luo L, Liu M. Adipose tissue in control of metabolism. The Journal of Endocrinology. 2016;**231**(3):R77-R99. DOI: 10.1530/JOE-16-0211

[47] Haylett WL, Ferris WF. Adipocyte-progenitor cell communication that influences adipogenesis. Cellular and Molecular Life Sciences. 2020;**77**(1):115-128. DOI: 10.1007/s00018-019-03256-5

[48] Harvey I, Boudreau A, Stephens JM. Adipose tissue in health and disease. Open Biology. 2020;**10**(12):200291. DOI: 10.1098/rsob.200291

[49] Longo M, Zatterale F, Naderi J, Parrillo L, Formisano P, et al. Adipose tissue dysfunction as determinant of obesity-associated metabolic complications. International Journal of Molecular Sciences. 2019;**20**(9):2358. DOI: 10.3390/ijms20092358

[50] Stenkula KG, Erlanson-Albertsson C. Adipose cell size: Importance in health and disease. American Journal of Physiology. Regulatory, Integrative and Comparative Physiology. 2018;**315**(2):R284-R295. DOI: 10.1152/ajpre gu.00257.2017

[51] Sun K, Kusminski CM, Scherer PE. Adipose tissue remodeling and obesity. The Journal of Clinical Investigation. 2011;**121**(6):2094-2101. DOI: 10.1172/JCI45887

[52] Liu R, Nikolajczyk BS. Tissue immune cells fuel obesity-associated inflammation in adipose tissue and beyond. Frontiers in Immunology. 2019;**10**:1587. DOI: 10.3389/fimmu.2019.01587

[53] Pan W, Myers M. Leptin and the maintenance of elevated body weight. Nature Reviews. Neuroscience. 2018;**19**:95-105. DOI: 10.1038/nrn.2017.168

[54] Zhang Y, Kilroy GE, Henagan TM, Prpic-Uhing V, Richards WG, Bannon AW, et al. Targeted deletion of melanocortin receptor subtypes 3 and 4, but not CART, alters nutrient partitioning and compromises behavioral and metabolic responses to leptin. The FASEB Journal. 2005;**19**(11):1482-1491. DOI: 10.1096/fj.05-3851com

[55] Wang ZV, Scherer PE. Adiponectin, the past two decades. Journal of Molecular Cell Biology. 2016;**8**(2):93-100. DOI: 10.1093/jmcb/mjw011

[56] Scheja L, Heeren J. The endocrine function of adipose tissues in health and cardiometabolic disease. Nature Reviews. Endocrinology. 2019;**15**(9):507-524. DOI: 10.1038/s41574-019-0230-6

[57] Karpe F, Pinnick KE. Biology of upper-body and lower-body adipose tissue—Link to whole-body phenotypes. Nature Reviews. Endocrinology. 2015;**11**(2):90-100. DOI: 10.1038/nrendo.2014.185

[58] Johnson D, Dixon AK, Abrahams PH. The abdominal subcutaneous tissue: Computed tomographic, magnetic resonance, and anatomical observations. Clinical Anatomy. 1996;**9**(1):19-24. DOI: 10.1002/(SICI)1098-2353(1996)9:1%3c19::AID-CA4%3e3.0.CO;2-V

[59] Kelley DE, Thaete FL, Troost F, Huwe T, Goodpaster BH. Subdivisions of subcutaneous abdominal adipose tissue and insulin resistance. American Journal of Physiological Metabolism. 2000;**278**(5):E941-E948. DOI: 10.1152/ajpendo.2000.278.5.E941

[60] Smith SR, Lovejoy JC, Greenway F, Ryan D, de Jonge L, de la Bretonne J, et al. Contributions of total body fat, abdominal subcutaneous adipose tissue compartments, and visceral adipose tissue to the metabolic complications of obesity. Metabolism. 2001;**50**(4):425-435. DOI: 10.1053/meta.2001.21693

[61] Golan R, Shelef I, Rudich A, Gepner Y, Shemesh E, Chassidim Y, et al. Abdominal superficial subcutaneous fat: A putative distinct protective fat subdepot in type 2 diabetes. Diabetes Care. 2012;**35**(3):640-647. DOI: 10.2337/dc11-1583

[62] Bjørndal B, Burri L, Staalesen V, Skorve J, Berge RK. Different adipose depots: Their role in the development of metabolic syndrome and mitochondrial response to hypolipidemic agents. Journal of Obesity. 2011;**2011**:490650. DOI: 10.1155/2011/490650

[63] Ibrahim MM. Subcutaneous and visceral adipose tissue: Structural and functional differences. Obesity Reviews. 2010;**11**(1):11-18. DOI: 10.1111/j.1467-789X.2009.00623.x

[64] Zhang W, Bi S. Hypothalamic regulation of brown adipose tissue thermogenesis and energy homeostasis. Frontiers in Endocrinology (Lausanne). 2015;**6**:136

[65] Ricquier D, Bouillaud F. Mitochondrial uncoupling proteins: From mitochondria to the regulation of energy balance. The Journal of Physiology. 2000;**529**(Pt1):3-10. DOI: 10.1111/j.1469-7793. 2000.00003.x

[66] Park A, Kim WK, Bae KH. Distinction of white, beige and brown adipocytes derived from mesenchymal stem cells. World Journal of Stem Cells. 2014;**6**(1):33-42. DOI: 10.4252/wjsc.v6.i1.33

[67] Lizcano F. The beige adipocyte as a therapy for metabolic diseases. International Journal of Molecular Sciences. 2019;**20**(20):5058. DOI: 10.3390/ijms20205058

[68] Cannon B, Nedergaard J. Brown adipose tissue: Function and physiological significance. Physiological Reviews. 2004;**84**(1):277-359. DOI: 10.1152/physrev.00015.2003

[69] Jastroch M, Oelkrug R, Keipert S. Insights into brown adipose tissue evolution and function from non-model organisms. Journal of Experimental Biology. 2018;**221** (Pt suppl 1):jeb169425

[70] Öztop M, Özbek M, Liman N, Beyaz F, Ergün E, Ergün L. Localization profiles of natriuretic peptides in hearts of pre-hibernating and hibernating Anatolian ground squirrels (*Spermophilus xanthoprymnus*). Veterinary Research Communications. 2019;**43**(2):45-65. DOI: 10.1007/s11259-019-9745-5

[71] Cypess AM, Lehman S, Williams G, Tal I, Rodman D, et al. Identification and importance of brown adipose tissue in adult humans. The New England Journal of Medicine. 2009;**360**(15):1509-1517. DOI: 10.1056/NEJMoa0810780

[72] Ouellet V, Labbé SM, Blondin DP, Phoenix S, Guérin B, Haman F, et al. Brown adipose tissue oxidative metabolism contributes to energy expenditure during acute cold exposure in humans. The Journal of Clinical Investigation. 2012;**122**(2):545-552. DOI: 10.1172/JCI60433

[73] Armani A, Infante M, Fabbri A, Caprio M. Comment on "mineralocorticoid antagonism enhances brown adipose tissue function in humans: A randomized placebo-controlled cross-over study". Diabetes, Obesity & Metabolism. 2019;**21**(8):2024-2026. DOI: 10.1111/dom.13756

[74] McNeill BT, Suchacki KJ, Stimson RH. Human brown adipose tissue as a therapeutic target: Warming up or cooling down? European Journal of Endocrinology. 2021;**184**(6):R243-R259. DOI: 10.1530/EJE-20-1439

[75] Virtanen KA, Lidell ME, Orava J, Heglind M, Westergren R, Niemi T, et al. Functional brown adipose tissue in healthy adults. The New England Journal of Medicine. 2009;**360**(15):1518-1525. DOI: 10.1056/NEJMoa0808949

[76] Orava J, Nuutila P, Noponen T, Parkkola R, Viljanen T, Enerbäck S, et al. Blunted metabolic responses to cold and insulin stimulation in brown adipose tissue of obese humans. Obesity (Silver Spring). 2013;**21**(11):2279-2287. DOI: 10.1002/oby.20456

[77] van der Lans AA, Hoeks J, Brans B, Vijgen GH, Visser MG, Vosselman MJ, et al. Cold acclimation recruits human brown fat and increases nonshivering thermogenesis. The Journal of Clinical Investigation. 2013;**123**(8):3395-3403. DOI: 10.1172/JCI68993

[78] Yoneshiro T, Aita S, Matsushita M, Kayahara T, Kameya T, Kawai Y, et al. Recruited brown adipose tissue as an anti-obesity agent in humans. The Journal of Clinical Investigation. 2013;**123**(8):3404-3408. DOI: 10.1172/JCI67803

[79] Blondin DP, Labbé SM, Tingelstad HC, Noll C, Kunach M, Phoenix S, et al. Increased brown adipose tissue oxidative capacity in cold-acclimated humans. The Journal of Clinical Endocrinology and Metabolism. 2014;**99**(3):E438-E446. DOI: 10.1210/jc.2013-3901

[80] Hanssen MJ, Hoeks J, Brans B, van der Lans AA, Schaart G, van den Driessche JJ, et al. Short-term cold acclimation improves insulin sensitivity in patients with type 2 diabetes mellitus. Nature Medicine. 2015;**21**(8):863-865. DOI: 10.1038/nm.3891

[81] Weir G, Ramage LE, Akyol M, Rhodes JK, Kyle CJ, Fletcher AM, et al. Substantial metabolic activity of human brown adipose tissue during warm conditions and cold-induced lipolysis of local triglycerides. Cell Metabolism. 2018;**27**(6):1348-1355

[82] Gunawardana SC, Piston DW. Reversal of type 1 diabetes in mice by brown adipose tissue transplant. Diabetes. 2012;**61**:674-682. DOI: 10.2337/db11-0510

[83] Gunawardana SC, Piston DW. Insulin-independent reversal of type 1 diabetes in nonobese diabetic mice with brown adipose tissue transplant. American Journal of Physiology. Endocrinology and Metabolism. 2015;**308**:E1043-E1055. DOI: 10.1152/ajpendo.00570.2014

[84] Gunawardana SC, Piston DW. Insulin-independent reversal of type-1 diabetes following transplantation of adult brown adipose tissue supplemented with IGF-1. Transplantation Direct. 2019;**5**(11):e500. DOI: 10.1097/TXD.0000000000000945

[85] Gunawardana SC, Infante M. Brown adipose tissue transplantation as a promising approach for insulin-independent reversal of type 1 diabetes: Animal studies and clinical perspectives. CellR4. 2020;**8**:e2986

[86] Aldiss P, Davies G, Woods R, Budge H, Sacks HS, et al. 'Browning' the cardiac and peri-vascular adipose tissues to modulate cardiovascular risk. International Journal of Cardiology. 2017;**228**:265-274. DOI: 10.1016/j.ijcard.2016.11.074

[87] Fitzgibbons TP, Czech MP. Epicardial and perivascular adipose tissues and their influence on cardiovascular disease: Basic mechanisms and clinical associations. Journal of American Heart Association. 2014;**3**:e000582

[88] Christensen RH, von Scholten BJ, Lehrskov LL, Rossing P, Jørgensen PG. Epicardial adipose tissue: An emerging biomarker of cardiovascular complications in type 2 diabetes? Therapeutic Advances in Endocrinology and Metabolism. 2020;**11**:1-16. DOI: 10.1177/2042018820928824

[89] Sacks HS, Fain JN, Bahouth SW, Ojha S, Frontini A, et al. Adult epicardial fat exhibits beige features. The Journal of Clinical Endocrinology and Metabolism. 2013;**98**(9):E1448-E1455. DOI: 10.1210/jc. 2013-1265

[90] Grigoras A, Amalinei C, Balan RA, Giusca SE, Caruntu ID. Perivascular adipose tissue in cardiovascular diseases-an update. Anatology Journal of Cardiology. 2019;**22**(5):219-231

[91] Koliaki C, Liatis S, Kokkinos A. Obesity and cardiovascular disease: Revisiting an old relationship. Metabolism. 2019;**92**:98-107. DOI: 10.1016/j.metabol.2018.10.011 65

[92] Lee HJ, Cantú SM, Álvarez Primo M, Peredo HA, Donoso AS, et al. Losartan prevents mesenteric vascular bed alterations in high-fat diet fed rats. Clínica e Investigación en Arteriosclerosis. 2021;**33**(1):1-9. DOI: 10.1016/j.arteri.2020.06.004

[93] Fuster JJ, Ouchi N, Gokce N, Walsh K. Obesity-induced changes in adipose tissue microenvironment

and their impact on cardiovascular disease. Circulation Research. 2016;**118**(11):1786-1807. DOI: 10.1161/CIRCRESAHA.115.306885

[94] Spalding KL, Arner E, Westermark PO, Bernard S, Buchholz BA, Bergmann O, et al. Dynamics of fat cell turnover in humans. Nature. 2008;**453**(7196):783-787. DOI: 10.1038/nature06902

[95] Rutkowski JM, Stern JH, Scherer PE. The cell biology of fat expansion. The Journal of Cell Biology. 2015;**208**(5):501-512. DOI: 10.1083/jcb.201409063

[96] Kabir M, Catalano KJ, Ananthnarayan S, Kim SP, Van Citters GW, Dea MK, et al. Molecular evidence supporting the portal theory: A causative link between visceral adiposity and hepatic insulin resistance. American Journal of Physiology. Endocrinology and Metabolism. 2005;**288**:E454-E461. DOI: 10.1152/ajpendo.00203.2004

[97] Item F, Konrad D. Visceral fat and metabolic inflammation: The portal theory revisited. Obesity Reviews. 2012;**13**(Suppl 2):30-39. DOI: 10.1111/j.1467-789X.2012.01035.x

[98] Jensen MD. Role of body fat distribution and the metabolic complications of obesity. The Journal of Clinical Endocrinology and Metabolism. 2008;**93**(11 Suppl 1):S57-S63. DOI: 10.1210/jc.2008-1585

[99] Bruun JM, Lihn AS, Pedersen SB, Richelsen B. Monocyte chemoattractant protein-1 release is higher in visceral than subcutaneous human adipose tissue (AT): Implication of macrophages resident in the AT. The Journal of Clinical Endocrinology and Metabolism. 2005;**90**(4):2282-2289. DOI: 10.1210/jc.2004-1696

[100] Park HS, Park JY, Yu R. Relationship of obesity and visceral adiposity with serum concentrations of CRP, TNF-alpha and IL-6. Diabetes Research and Clinical Practice. 2005;**69**(1):29-35. DOI: 10.1016/j.diabres.2004.11.007

[101] Boucher J, Kleinridders A, Kahn CR. Insulin receptor signaling in normal and insulin-resistant states. Cold Spring Harbor Perspectives in Biology. 2014;**6**(1):a009191. DOI: 10.1101/cshperspect.a009191

[102] Mancuso P. The role of adipokines in chronic inflammation. Immunotargets Therapeutics. 2016;**5**:47-56. DOI: 10.2147/ITT.S73223

[103] Haase J, Weyer U, Immig K, Klöting N, Blüher M, et al. Local proliferation of macrophages in adipose tissue during obesity-induced inflammation. Diabetologia. 2014;**57**(3):562-571. DOI: 10.1007/s00125-013-3139-y

[104] Lihn AS, Bruun JM, He G, Pedersen SB, Jensen PF, et al. Lower expression of adiponectin mRNA in visceral adipose tissue in lean and obese subjects. Molecular and Cellular Endocrinology. 2004;**219**(1-2):9-15. DOI: 10.1016/j.mce.2004.03.002

[105] Gustafson B, Smith U. Regulation of white adipogenesis and its relation to ectopic fat accumulation and cardiovascular risk. Atherosclerosis. 2015;**241**(1):27-35. DOI: 10.1016/j.atherosclerosis.2015.04.812

[106] Fabbrini E, Magkos F, Mohammed BS, Pietka T, Abumrad NA, et al. Intrahepatic fat, not visceral fat, is linked with metabolic complications of obesity. Proceedings of the National Academy of Science USA. 2009;**106**(36):15430-15435. DOI: 10.1073/pnas.0904944106

[107] Ketonen J, Shi J, Martonen E, Mervaala E. Periadventitial adipose

tissue promotes endothelial dysfunction via oxidative stress in diet-induced obese C57Bl/6 mice. Circulation Journal. 2010;**74**(7):147914-147987. DOI: 10.1253/circj.cj-09-0661

[108] Qi XY, Qu SL, Xiong WH, Rom O, Chang L, et al. Perivascular adipose tissue (PVAT) in atherosclerosis: A double-edged sword. Cardiovascular Diabetology. 2018;**17**(1):134. DOI: 10.1186/s12933-018-0777-x

[109] DeFronzo RA. Pathogenesis of type 2 diabetes mellitus. The Medical Clinics of North America. 2004;**88**:787-835. DOI: 10.1016/j.mcna.2004.04.013

[110] Abel ED, Peroni O, Kim JK, Kim Y-B, Boss O, Hadro E, et al. Adipose-selective targeting of the GLUT4 gene impairs insulin action in muscle and liver. Nature. 2001;**409**:729-733. DOI: 10.1038/35055575

[111] Blüher M, Michael MD, Peroni OD, Ueki K, Carter N, Kahn BB, et al. Adipose tissue selective insulin receptor knockout protects against obesity and obesity-related glucose intolerance. Developmental Cell. 2002;**3**:25-38. DOI: 10.1016/S1534-5807(02)00199-5

[112] Sakaguchi M, Fujisaka S, Cai W, Winnay JN, Konishi M, O'Neill BT, et al. Adipocyte dynamics and reversible metabolic syndrome in mice with an inducible adipocyte-specific deletion of the insulin receptor. Cell Metabolism. 2017;**25**(2):448-462. DOI: 10.1016/j.cmet.2016.12.008

[113] Morigny P, Houssier M, Mouisel E, Langin D. Adipocyte lipolysis and insulin resistance. Biochimie. 2016;**125**:259-266. DOI: 10.1016/j.biochi.2015.10.024

[114] Cawthorn WP, Sethi JK. TNF-α and adipocyte biology. FEBS Letters. 2008;**582**:117-131. DOI: 10.1016/j.febslet.2007.11.051

[115] Frühbeck G, Méndez-Giménez L, Fernández-Formoso J-A, Fernández S, Rodríguez A. Regulation of adipocyte lipolysis. Nutrition Research Reviews. 2014;**27**:63-93. DOI: 10.1017/S095442241400002X

[116] Rockall AG, Sohaib SA, Evans D, Kaltsas G, Isidori AM, Monson JP, et al. Hepatic steatosis in Cushing's syndrome: A radiological assessment using computed tomography. European Journal of Endocrinology. 2003;**149**:543-548. DOI: 10.1530/eje.0.1490543

[117] Scaroni C, Zilio M, Foti M, Boscaro M. Glucose metabolism abnormalities in Cushing syndrome: From molecular basis to clinical management. Endocrine Reviews. 2017;**38**:189-219. DOI: 10.1210/er.2016-1105

[118] Gavrilova O, Marcus-Samuels B, Graham D, Kim JK, Shulman GI, Castle AL, et al. Surgical implantation of adipose tissue reverses diabetes in lipoatrophic mice. The Journal of Clinical Investigation. 2000;**105**:271-278. DOI: 10.1172/JCI7901

[119] Moreno-Santos I, Macías-González M, Porras-Martín C, Castellano-Castillo D, Sánchez-Espín G, et al. Role of epicardial adipose tissue NPR-C in acute coronary syndrome. Atherosclerosis. 2019;**286**:79-87. DOI: 10.1016/j.atherosclerosis.2019. 05.010

[120] Garruti G, Giusti V, Nussberger J, Darimont C, Verdumo C, et al. Expression and secretion of the atrial natriuretic peptide in human adipose tissue and preadipocytes. Obesity (Silver Spring). 2007;**15**(9):2181-2189. DOI: 10.1038/oby.2007.259

[121] Katafuchi T, Garbers DL, Albanesi JP. CNP/GC-B system: A new regulator of adipogenesis. Peptides.

2010;**31**(10):1906-1911. DOI: 10.1016/j.peptides.2010.06.025

[122] Bae CR, Hino J, Hosoda H, Arai Y, Son C, et al. Overexpression of C-type peptide in endothelial cells protects against insulin resistance and inflammation during diet-induced obesity. Scientific Reports. 2017;7(1):9807. DOI: 10.1038/s41598-017-10240-1

[123] Moro C, Lafontan M. Natriuretic peptides and cGMP signaling control of energy homeostasis. American Journal of Physiology. Heart and Circulatory Physiology. 2013;**304**(3):H358-H368. DOI: 10.1152/ajphe art.00704.2012

[124] Shi F, Simandi Z, Nagy L, Collins S. Diet-dependent natriuretic peptide receptor C expression in adipose tissue is mediated by PPARγ via long-range distal enhancers. The Journal of Biological Chemistry. 2021;**297**(2):100941. DOI: 10.1016/j.jbc.2021.100941

[125] Fain JN, Kanu A, Bahouth SW, Cowan GS, Lloyd HM. Inhibition of leptin release by atrial natriuretic peptide (ANP) in human adipocytes. Biochemical Pharmacology. 2003;**65**(11):1883-1888. DOI: 10.1016/s0006-2952(03)00154-0

[126] Tsukamoto O, Fujita M, Kato M, Yamazaki S, Asano Y, et al. Natriuretic peptides enhance the production of adiponectin in human adipocytes and in patients with chronic heart failure. Journal of the American College of Cardiology. 2009;**53**(22):2070-2077. DOI: 10.1016/j. jacc.2009.02.038

[127] Bordicchia M, Liu D, Amri EZ, Ailhaud G, Dessì-Fulgheri P, et al. Cardiac natriuretic peptides act via p38 MAPK to induce the brown fat thermogenic program in mouse and human adipocytes. Journal of the Clinical Investment. 2012;**122**(3):1022-1036

[128] Palmer BF, Clegg DJ. An emerging role of natriuretic peptides: Igniting the fat furnace to fuel and warm the heart. Mayo Clinic Proceedings. 2015;**90**(12):1666-1678. DOI: 10.1016/j.mayocp.2015.08.006

[129] Carper D, Coué M, Nascimento EBM, Barquissau V, Lagarde D, et al. Atrial natriuretic peptide orchestrates a coordinated physiological response to fuel non-shivering thermogenesis. Cell Reports. 2020;**32**(8):108075. DOI: 10.1016/j.celrep.2020.108075

[130] Galitzky J, Sengenès C, Thalamas C, Marques MA, Senard JM, et al. The lipid-mobilizing effect of atrial natriuretic peptide is unrelated to sympathetic nervous system activation or obesity in young men. Journal of Lipid Research. 2001;**42**(4):536-544. DOI: 10.1016/S0022-2275(20)31162-7

[131] Kalra PR, Tigas S. Regulation of lipolysis: Natriuretic peptides and the development of cachexia. International Journal of Cardiology. 2002;**85**(1):125-132. DOI: 10.1016/s0167-5273(02)00241-3

[132] Niessner A, Ziegler S, Slany J, Billensteiner E, Woloszczuk W, et al. Increases in plasma levels of atrial and brain natriuretic peptides after running a marathon: Are their effects partly counterbalanced by adrenocortical steroids? European Journal of Endocrinology. 2003;**149**(6):555-559. DOI: 10.1530/eje.0.1490555

[133] Birkenfeld AL, Boschmann M, Engeli S, Moro C, Arafat AM, et al. Atrial natriuretic peptide and adiponectin interactions in man. PLoS One. 2012;7(8):e43238. DOI: 10.1371/journal.pone.0043238

[134] Tanaka T, Tsutamoto T, Sakai H, Nishiyama K, Fujii M, Yamamoto T,

et al. Effect of atrial natriuretic peptide on adiponectin in patients with heart failure. European Journal of Heart Failure. 2008;**10**(4):360-366. DOI: 10.1016/j.ejheart.2008.02.005

[135] Cabiati M, Raucci S, Liistro T, Belcastro E, Prescimone T, et al. Impact of obesity on the expression profile of natriuretic peptide system in a rat experimental model. PLoS One. 2013;**8**(8):e72959. DOI: 10.1371/journal.pone.0072959

[136] Plante E, Menaouar A, Danalache BA, Broderick TL, Jankowski M, et al. Treatment with brain natriuretic peptide prevents the development of cardiac dysfunction in obese diabetic db/db mice. Diabetologia. 2014;**57**(6):1257-1267. DOI: 10.1007/s00125-014-3201-4

[137] Coué M, Badin PM, Vila IK, Laurens C, Louche K, et al. Defective natriuretic peptide receptor signaling in skeletal muscle links obesity to type 2 diabetes. Diabetes. 2015;**64**(12):4033-4045. DOI: 10.2337/db15-0305

[138] Standeven KF, Hess K, Carter AM, Rice GI, Cordell PA, et al. Neprilysin, obesity and the metabolic syndrome. International Journal of Obesity. 2011;**35**(8):1031-1340. DOI: 10.1038/ijo.2010.227

[139] Mehra MR, Uber PA, Park MH, Scott RL, Ventura HO, et al. Obesity and suppressed B-type natriuretic peptide levels in heart failure. Journal of the American College of Cardiology. 2004;**43**(9):1590-1595. DOI: 10.1016/j.jacc.2003.10.066

[140] Wang TJ, Larson MG, Levy D, Benjamin EJ, Leip EP, et al. Impact of obesity on plasma natriuretic peptide levels. Circulation. 2004;**109**:594-600. DOI: 10.1161/01.CIR.0000112582.16683.EA

[141] Neeland IJ, Winders BR, Ayers CR, Das SR, Chang AY, et al. Higher natriuretic peptide levels associate with a favorable adipose tissue distribution profile. Journal of the American College of Cardiology. 2013;**62**(8):752-760. DOI: 10.1016/j.jacc.2013.03.038

[142] Kovacova Z, Tharp WG, Liu D, Wei W, Xie H, et al. Adipose tissue natriuretic peptide receptor expression is related to insulin sensitivity in obesity and diabetes. Obesity (Silver Spring). 2016;**24**(4):820-828. DOI: 10.1002/oby.21418

[143] Seferovic JP, Solomon SD, Seely EW. Potential mechanisms of beneficial effect of sacubitril/valsartan on glycemic control. Therapeutic Advances. 2020, 2020;**11**:1-9

[144] Wu W, Shi F, Liu D, Ceddia RP, Gaffin R, et al. Enhancing natriuretic peptide signaling in adipose tissue, but not in muscle, protects against diet-induced obesity and insulin resistance. Science Signalling. 2017;**10**(489):eaam6870

[145] Oliver PM, Fox JE, Kim R, Rockman HA, Kim HS, et al. Hypertension, cardiac hypertrophy, and sudden death in mice lacking natriuretic peptide receptor A. Proceedings of the National Academy of Science USA. 1997;**94**(26):14730-14735. DOI: 10.1073/pnas.94.26.14730

[146] Miyashita K, Itoh H, Tsujimoto H, Tamura N, Fukunaga Y, et al. Natriuretic peptides/cGMP/cGMP-dependent protein kinase cascades promote muscle mitochondrial biogenesis and prevent obesity. Diabetes. 2009;**58**:2880-2892. DOI: 10.2337/db09-0393

[147] Bae CR, Hino J, Hosoda H, Son C, Makino H, et al. Adipocyte-specific

expression of C-type natriuretic peptide suppresses lipid metabolism and adipocyte hypertrophy in adipose tissues in mice fed high-fat diet. Scientific Reports. 2018;**8**(1):2093. DOI: 10.1038/s41598-018-20469-z

[148] Chavez JA, Summers SA. A ceramide-centric view of insulin resistance. Cell Metabolism. 2012;**15**:585-594. DOI: 10.1016/j.cmet.2012.04.002

[149] Samuel VT, Shulman GI. Mechanisms for insulin resistance: Common threads and missing links. Cell. 2012;**148**:852-871. DOI: 10.1016/j.cell.2012.02.017

[150] Pivovarova O, Gögebakan Ö, Klöting N, et al. Insulin up-regulates natriuretic peptide clearance receptor expression in the subcutaneous fat depot in obese subjects: A missing link between CVD risk and obesity? The Journal of Clinical Endocrinology and Metabolism. 2012;**97**:E731-E739. DOI: 10.1210/jc.2011-2839

[151] Sarzani R, Dessì-Fulgheri P, Salvi F, et al. A novel promoter variant of the natriuretic peptide clearance receptor gene is associated with lower atrial natriuretic peptide and higher blood pressure in obese hypertensives. Journal of Hypertension. 1999;**17**:1301-1305. DOI: 10.1097/00004872-199917090-00010

[152] Sarzani R, Strazzullo P, Salvi F, et al. Natriuretic peptide clearance receptor alleles and susceptibility to abdominal adiposity. Obesity Research. 2004;**12**:351-356. DOI: 10.1038/oby.2004.44

[153] Khan AM, Cheng S, Magnusson M, et al. Cardiac natriuretic peptides, obesity, and insulin resistance: Evidence from two community-based studies. The Journal of Clinical Endocrinology and Metabolism. 2011;**96**:3242-3249. DOI: 10.1210/jc.2011-1182

[154] Matsukawa N, Grzesik WJ, Takahashi N, et al. The natriuretic peptide clearance receptor locally modulates the physiological effects of the natriuretic peptide system. Proceedings of the National Academy of Science USA. 1999;**96**:7403-7408. DOI: 10.1073/pnas.96.13.7403

Chapter 7

Berardinelli-Seip Syndrome: Report of an Old Case Successfully Treated with Anti-Glucocorticoid Therapy Followed by Bilateral Adrenalectomy

Patricio H. Contreras

Abstract

A female teenager was diagnosed in 1986 with Berardinelli-Seip syndrome (congenital generalized lipodystrophy). Following the predictable failure of the usual treatments for her severe type 2 diabetes and hypertriglyceridemia, we decided to treat her with a novel anti-glucocorticoid-centered approach. In 1988, we treated her with mifepristone alone (9 weeks), then with mifepristone combined with ketoconazole (1 week), and again, with mifepristone alone (2 weeks). Acanthosis nigricans, as well as eruptive xanthomas, experienced complete regression following the anti-glucocorticoid therapy. Moreover, the patient gained 7 kilograms. Besides, there was a striking metabolic amelioration with mifepristone therapy. The addition of ketoconazole strongly reduced the relevant mifepristone-induced hypercortisolemia within 1 week. Fasting serum glucose, insulin, and triglycerides fell from day 1 to day 7 without reaching values within the normal range. Two weeks after ketoconazole withdrawal (while keeping mifepristone administration), serum triglyceride and glucose values rose significantly. Eleven days after bilateral adrenalectomy, fasting glucose values were within normal limits or slightly above. An oral glucose tolerance test (75-g OGTT) performed 13 days after surgery showed insulin values within normal limits, fasting serum glucose values within the normal range, and a 2-h serum glucose value in the diabetic range. These findings were consistent with our working hypothesis proposing that Berardinelli-Seip syndrome is due to cortisol-mediated unrestrained lipolysis.

Keywords: Berardinelli-Seip syndrome, hypoleptinemia, hypothalamic–pituitary–adrenal-axis overactivity, unrestrained lipolysis, mifepristone, ketoconazole

1. Introduction

Congenital Generalized Lipodystrophy (CGL, Berardinelli-Seip syndrome, BSCL) is a rare autosomal recessive disorder with a prevalence in the range of 1–10 patients per million people [1, 2]. However, in northern areas of Brazil, its prevalence is much higher, amounting to 32.3 patients per million people [3]. We recognize at least four CGL types: Type 1, due to mutations in the AGPAT2 gene, which is located on chromosome 9q34 and encodes the enzyme 1-acylglycerol-3-phosphate O-acyltransferase 2 (AGPAT2); Type 2, due to mutations in the BSCL2 gene, which is located on chromosome 11q13 and encodes Seipin; Type 3, due to mutations in the CAV1 gene, which is located on chromosome 7q31 and encodes caveolin-1; and Type 4, due to mutations in the polymerase I and transcript-release factor [PTRF] gene, which is located on chromosome 17q21.2 and encodes cavin [1].

About 95% of CGL patients harbor either AGPAT2 or seipin mutations. The most common CGL is Type 1, and the rarest is Type 3. In Brazil, over 90% of CGL cases are CGL type 2, while in Europe, Middle East, and Japan, most patients have CGL Type 1. CGL patients have an extreme deficiency of fat depots. Therefore, most CGL patients have low serum leptin and adiponectin levels. They usually have elevated circulating serum triglycerides (very-low-density lipoproteins plus chylomicrons) and develop severe steatosis within their lean organs, such as the liver and skeletal muscles. Lipotoxicity of these organs produces in CGL patients an insulin-resistant state that does not respond to current treatments.

Two key metabolic features are prominent in these patients: much-elevated gluconeogenesis along with much-reduced insulin-mediated skeletal muscle glucose uptake. Usually, by the second decade of life, these patients develop type 2 diabetes requiring very high insulin doses. Hypertriglyceridemia in these patients is very difficult to treat, and it may manifest itself as cutaneous xanthomas. The best current treatment for CGL is recombinant leptin [4], but this is not widely available. Besides, leptin therapy is associated with weight loss in these patients.

The first two reported patients—both of pediatric age—were described in Brazil by Dr. Waldemar Berardinelli in 1954 [5]. In 1959, the Norwegian pediatrician Martin Seip published the report of three additional patients [6]. Berardinelli-Seip syndrome has been hard to understand and therefore, very difficult to treat.

To advance the knowledge on CGL, several groups attempted to generate transgenic murine models of the disease. In 1998, two transgenic models of murine lipoatrophy were simultaneously published [7, 8]. The A-ZIP/F1 transgenic mouse model had an extreme fat deficiency, whereas the aP2-SREBP-1c mouse model had only a moderate fat deficiency.

In 1994, leptin (a cytokine produced by the adipocytes having endocrine actions) was discovered [9]. In 1999, Shimomura et al. [10] showed that recombinant leptin reversed diabetes in the aP2-SREBP-1c mouse model of CGL and concluded that insulin resistance was secondary to the severe hypoleptinemia found in these animals. However, the A-ZIP/F1 mouse model responded poorly to exogenous leptin [11]. By contrast, in 2002, a study demonstrated that total adrenalectomy in A-ZIP/F1 diabetic mice induced a substantial metabolic improvement by increasing liver and muscle insulin sensitivity [12]. The authors attributed these improvements to the adrenalectomy-induced disappearance of chronic hypercorticosteronemia. Moreover, leptin treatment in A-ZIP/F1 mice reduced their elevated circulating corticosterone levels. So, it was conceivable that hypoleptinemia was behind the adrenal axis overactivation and the subsequent hypercorticosteronemic state exhibited by this mouse model.

In 2002, recombinant methionyl human leptin (metreleptin) reversed insulin resistance in nine women with congenital or acquired lipodystrophy and serum leptin levels <4 ng/mL [4]. In 2014, recombinant human leptin (metreleptin; Myalept®) received FDA approval to treat lipodystrophies [13]. In 2009, Cortés et al. generated the AGPAT2-deficient mouse, a transgenic animal model of lipoatrophy resembling CGL Type 1 [14]. In 2011, Cui et al. [15] reported that seipin ablation in mice results in severe generalized lipodystrophy. In 2012, Chen et al. [16] confirmed that inactivation of seipin in mice leads to severe lipodystrophy. Also, these authors shed light on the mechanisms involved in the process. They found that in vitro differentiation of murine embryonic fibroblast and stromal vascular cells had normal early-phase adipocyte differentiation, but a striking failure of terminal differentiation. This unsuccessful adipogenesis was secondary to a runaway cyclic AMP-dependent lipolysis and silencing of the transcription factors regulating adipogenesis. In vitro adipogenesis was rescued by inhibitors of lipolysis, but not by peroxisome proliferator-activated receptor (PPAR)-gamma agonists, such as pioglitazone. A recent review [17] suggests a central role of unrestrained lipolysis in the genesis of lipoatrophy of seipin-deficient individuals. In summary, seipin stimulates adipogenesis and inhibits cyclic AMP-dependent lipolysis.

The pathophysiology of the AGPAT2-deficient patients is cloudier compared with the situation of the homologous seipin-deficient patients. In 2016, Cautivo et al. [18] showed that the AGPAT2 gene is essential for the postnatal development and maintenance of white and brown adipose tissue.

A simplistic belief is that AGPAT2 deficiency impairs lipogenesis, while seipin deficiency impairs normal adipogenesis. Both conditions result in triglyceride (TG)-depleted adipocytes. However, a TG-depleted adipocyte also results from ablation of perilipin in murine adipose tissue. Nevertheless, in the latter situation, the TG-depleted adipocyte secretes an increased, rather than a reduced, amount of leptin [19]. Thus, a TG-depleted adipocyte is not necessarily associated with hypoleptinemia. In other words, the exact mechanism by which AGPAT2 deficiency leads to hypoleptinemia is unknown. Overall, hypoleptinemia seems to be a commonality in generalized lipodystrophies. Therefore, the biggest investigational challenge is to figure out how hypoleptinemia and severe insulin resistance are linked together in CGL.

Herein, we report an extraordinary experience with a patient with Berardinelli-Seip syndrome (1986–1988) seen before the leptin era. At that time, we hypothesized that CGL was somehow the consequence of the local excess of cortisol action on the adipocyte. To test our daring hypothesis, we used mifepristone, a potent anti-glucocorticoid drug. Having previous experience with the drug on a patient with a previously operated-on, recurrent ectopic adrenal cancer and severe Cushing's syndrome [20], we anticipated that mifepristone would probably produce an overactivation of the hypothalamic–pituitary–adrenal axis. For this reason, following 9 weeks of mifepristone therapy alone, we briefly added ketoconazole to the treatment to partially block cortisol synthesis. We devised this therapeutic strategy to reduce serum cortisol levels, seeking to reinforce the anti-glucocorticoid effect of mifepristone. Finally, we stopped ketoconazole to reduce the anti-glucocorticoid action of the combined intervention. Overall, our results with the abovementioned anti-glucocorticoid approach permitted us to surmise that total adrenalectomy would benefit the patient.

1.1 Case report

A 16-year-old female patient entered the Endocrine Unit of the University Hospital (Hospital José Joaquín Aguirre, Universidad de Chile, Santiago) with a recent diagnosis of type 2 diabetes. Her parents were first cousins. Since she was born, pediatricians were intrigued by her peculiar appearance, characterized by scarcity of subcutaneous fat, muscular prominence, and abdominal distension.

Our patient had an acromegaloid face, scarcity of subcutaneous adipose tissue, conservation of mechanical fat, severe acanthosis nigricans, prominent veins, and muscular prominence. She had a voracious appetite and exhibited eruptive xanthomas (sparing the face and the chest) especially over her palms and elbows.

She also had clinical hyperandrogenism, including facial and scalp seborrhea and mild clitoromegaly. She had a history of recurrent periods of amenorrhea. Her liver and spleen were notoriously enlarged, producing a prominent abdomen. A mild thyromegaly and a small umbilical hernia were present. The normal intellectual development and the presence of mechanical fat (located in palms, soles, joints, and retro-orbital space) in our patient suggested that she was AGPAT2-deficient rather than seipin-deficient. We did not have her DNA sequenced since this technique debuted in CGL cases just in the current century.

Fasting serum glucose, insulin, and triglycerides were 225 mg/dL, >400 mU/L, and 7400 mg/dL, respectively (normal levels: ≤99 mg/dL, ≤13 mU/L, and ≤ 150 mg/dL, respectively). The patient was diagnosed with Berardinelli-Seip syndrome and polycystic ovary syndrome.

We treated her with high insulin doses with disappointing results, which attested to the presence of an extreme insulin resistance. Given the acute pancreatitis risk, we carried out an unsuccessful attempt to reduce her extremely high levels of serum triglycerides with high doses of omega-3-rich fish oil (up to 20 grams per day). Our medical staff thoroughly discussed the case and reached a consensus: she was not treatable with conventional medications.

1.2 Rethinking the patient from scratch

We realized that, to help the patient, we had to rethink her. For us, the extreme scarcity of body fat in our patient was the key to understanding how to deal with her disease. We reviewed the available literature (years 1986–1988) regarding adipogenesis, lipogenesis, and lipolysis. We looked at the fat storage within the adipocyte like a "bank account" of fat. An "empty adipocyte" could result from deficient lipogenesis or increased lipolysis.

We learned that serum insulin levels stimulate lipoprotein lipase (LPL). LPL provokes the lipolysis of circulating serum chylomicrons and very-low-density lipoprotein particles (VLDL). Then, free fatty acid (FFA) molecules enter the adipocyte to initiate lipogenesis. Three FFA molecules bind to a single acyl-glycerol molecule to form the triacylglycerol molecule (triglyceride or TG) stored within lipid droplets inside the cytoplasm. The stored TG molecule may be subjected to a hormone-sensitive lipase (HSL)-mediated lipolysis, releasing FFAs and glycerol into the circulation. Even minute amounts of circulating insulin can tonically inhibit HSL.

When hepatic glycogenolysis is exhausted at dawn, serum glucose and insulin levels fall, interrupting the HSL inhibition. For us, a piece of crucial information was that cortisol exerts a permissive role on the HSL activation in the cytosol of the adipocyte. In other words, the HSL is inactive in the absence of cortisol inside the cytosol of the adipocyte. Cortisol reaches the cytosol of the adipocyte through the internalization of extracellular, inactive cortisone. This inactive cortisone is transformed inside the cytosol into physiologically active cortisol by the enzyme 11β-hydroxysteroid dehydrogenase type 1 (11β-HSD1). In turn, cortisol stimulates HSL acutely, whereas it stimulates LPL chronically. Acute lipolysis occurs when energy is required: the released FFA and glycerol molecules provide the liver with substrates to increase glucose production at dawn. These tips summarize what we learned about lipogenesis and lipolysis by reviewing the available literature. By understanding the physiological roles of leptin, our comprehension of adipose tissue physiology has grown a great deal. This new knowledge will allow us to reinterpret our extraordinary findings.

1.3 The decision to initiate an anti-glucocorticoid-centered, experimental therapeutic approach

Theoretically, fat depletion in CGL may be secondary to defects either in adipogenesis or lipogenesis. However, other possibilities may exist. We hypothesized that cortisol-mediated, unrestrained lipolysis was at the core of the CGL in our patient.

The main advantage of our daring—and even naïve—hypothesis was its testability. Serendipitously, we did have access to mifepristone (RU-486), a potent anti-progesterone and anti-glucocorticoid steroidal drug. We had previously treated with mifepristone for 5 months a patient with recurrent hepatic adrenal rest cancer-mediated hypercortisolism. Before that experience, back in 1985, we had postulated in a Lancet letter [21] that glucocorticoid-producing adrenal cancers might be glucocorticoid-dependent. We had observed a striking, rapid disappearance of liver and lung metastases after using ketoconazole (1200 mg/day) on a female patient to block excessive cortisol synthesis by adrenal cancer. Roussel-Uclaf kindly donated 1000 pills of mifepristone (200 mg each) to treat this patient with an ectopic adrenal cancer. That trial taught us what to expect from the mifepristone administration. However, when the hypercortisolism spectacularly faded away after 5 months of treatment, the patient declared herself cured, refusing further treatment. Unfortunately, she died less than a year after stopping treatment. We, therefore, were left with a substantial amount of available mifepristone pills.

Also, we had extensive experience with ketoconazole in several cases of Cushing's syndrome (seen from 1983 through 1988). In 1983, we successfully used ketoconazole to treat hypercortisolism in a patient with an adrenal rest tumor of the liver. This success permitted us to remove her ectopic adrenal tumor from the liver, resulting in an apparent surgical cure. We reported this experience in 1985 [20]. Up until then, nobody else had published a clinical trial with ketoconazole in Cushing's syndrome. This initial, positive experience paved the way for us to acquire expertise in using ketoconazole in Cushing's syndrome.

The endocrinologists of our Unit discussed the complex situation of our patient with CGL. At the time, we did not have an Ethics Committee at the University Hospital. Therefore, our group reached a medical consensus: to offer an experimental mifepristone treatment to the patient and her family. We explained to them that we had nothing else to offer. The patient and her family agreed to receive a trial of mifepristone therapy. We used the same dose of mifepristone (600 mg daily, divided into three 200 mg pills) that we had previously used in our patient with ectopic adrenal cancer. So, after a whole year of unsuccessful therapies, we were ready to proceed with an experimental, unheard-of, therapeutic approach on our 18-year-old patient.

2. Material and methods

2.1 Experimental protocol (1988)

2.1.1 First course of anti-glucocorticoid treatment alone

Mifepristone therapy alone (600 mg/day, given as three 200-mg pills, at 7 AM, 3 PM, and 11 PM) was administered orally for 9 weeks. The anti-glucocorticoid action of the drug would negate the cortisol-mediated negative feedback on secretion of CRF (corticotropin releasing factor) and ACTH (adrenocorticotropic hormone). Therefore, we anticipated an overactive hypothalamic–pituitary–adrenal axis ("adrenal axis", for short). High circulating cortisol levels will not produce glucocorticoid actions in the presence of mifepristone. Instead, they will stimulate the mineralocorticoid receptor in the distal renal tubule (cortisol-induced hypermineralocortisolism).

For this reason, we measured the mean daily serum cortisol values (individual values were measured at 8 AM, 3 PM, and 11 PM) and urinary free cortisol on day 63 of the trial at the end of this first phase. To monitor the expected metabolic changes, we serially measured serum fasting glucose, insulin, and triglycerides during this period.

2.1.2 Anti-glucocorticoid treatment plus partial blockade of cortisol synthesis

Mifepristone (600 mg/day) plus ketoconazole (800 mg/day, divided into four 200-mg pills given every 6 hours) combination therapy was administered for 1 week.

Ketoconazole was expected to produce a partial blockade of the enhanced mifepristone-induced adrenal cortisol synthesis, thus reducing the prevailing

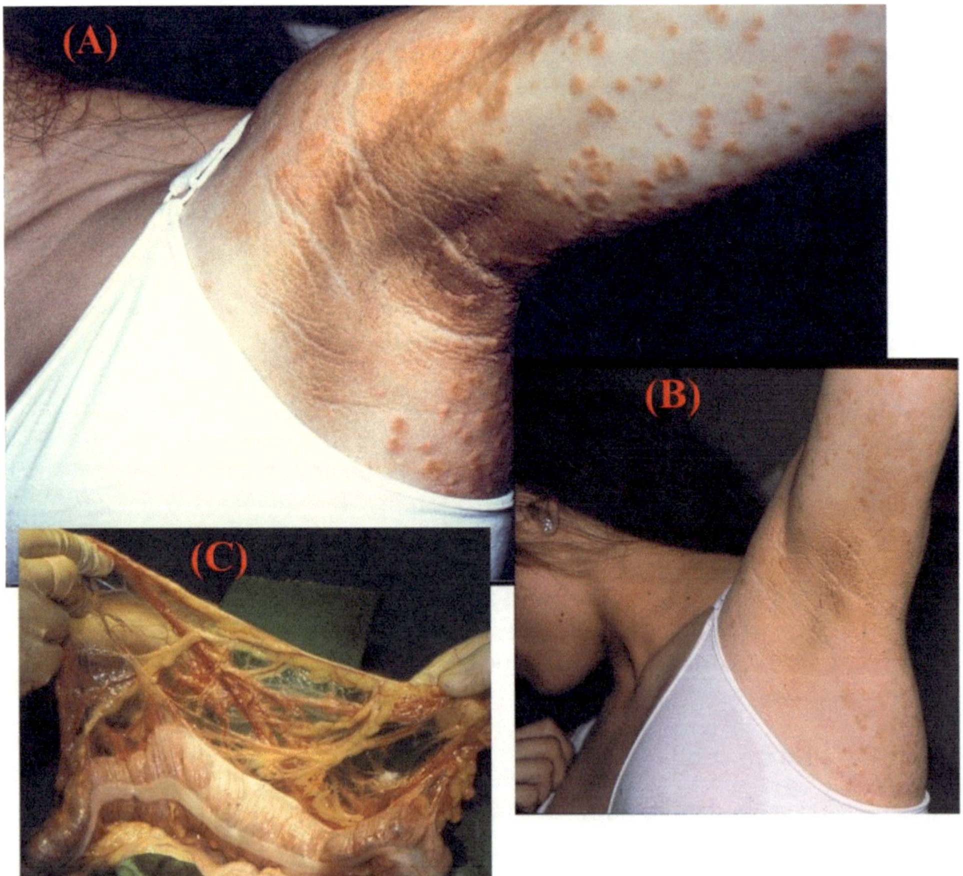

Figure 1.
Local acanthosis nigricans and eruptive xanthomas, as seen before (A) and after (B) the anti-glucocorticoid intervention. The peculiar aspect of a fat-devoid mesentery at surgery is also shown (C).

hypercortisolemia. We devised this therapeutic addition to reinforce the anti-glucocorticoid effect of mifepristone. We measured the daily mean serum cortisol values and urinary free cortisol on day 70 of the trial, at the end of the second phase of treatment. We also measured daily serum fasting glucose, insulin, and triglycerides to evaluate the response to the addition of ketoconazole.

2.1.3 Second course of anti-glucocorticoid treatment alone

Mifepristone therapy alone (600 mg/day, given as 200-mg pills, at 7 AM, 3 PM, and 11 PM) was administered orally for 2 weeks. We expected to witness a deterioration of both circulating fasting glucose and triglycerides by stopping ketoconazole. We did not measure cortisol values in serum and urine during this phase.

The whole anti-glucocorticoid intervention (mifepristone alone or combined with ketoconazole) lasted 12 weeks. Acanthosis nigricans and eruptive xanthomas virtually disappeared during the trial (**Figure 1**). Moreover, the patient gained 7 kilograms.

3. Results

3.1 Mifepristone therapy alone, 600 mg/day (9 weeks)

This intervention produced a striking amelioration of fasting serum insulin and triglyceride levels, as shown in **Table 1**. However, as we predicted, the patient experienced an overactivation of the adrenal axis, reflected by very high daily mean serum cortisol and urinary free cortisol excretion at the end of the 9th week (**Table 2**). The mifepristone-induced adrenal axis overactivity revealed itself as a clinical hypermineralocortisolism. The patient had arterial hypertension (160/100 mmHg), hypokalemia (3.4 mEq/L), and inappropriate urinary potassium loss (56 mEq/day).

Weeks	Serum fasting triglycerides (mg/dL)	Fasting glycemia (mg/dL)	Fasting insulinemia (mU/L)
Baseline	7400	225	>400
Week 1	6310	145	>400
Week 2	3625	250	10.0
Week 3	1220	280	20.0
Week 4	1210	230	18.0
Week 5	1200	290	n/a
Week 6	1500	230	10.0
Week 7	1750	225	11.0
Week 8	1500	224	10.5
Week 9	617	227	8.0

Table 1.
Assessment of metabolic parameters at baseline and after initiation of mifepristone therapy alone (600 mg/day). Mifepristone alone (600 mg/day) reduced serum triglycerides first (1 week) and then reduced serum fasting insulin levels in 2 weeks. Serum fasting glucose levels were unchanged for 9 weeks. At the end of the 9th week, serum levels of triglycerides were just 8.3% of the baseline value. Similarly, fasting insulin levels were less than 2% of the baseline value. Abbreviations: n/a, not available.

Intervention	24-hour urinary-free cortisol (UFC) (mcg/24 h; normal values, ≤100)	Mean daily serum cortisol* (mcg/dL)
Mifepristone therapy alone (63rd day)	1130	48.5
Mifepristone plus ketoconazole combination therapy (70th day)	630	26

Table 2.
*Assessment of adrenal function at the end of the prolonged mifepristone therapy alone and at the end of the mifepristone plus ketoconazole combination therapy. At the end of the administration of mifepristone alone, 24-h urinary free cortisol (UFC) and mean daily serum cortisol values were grossly elevated, reflecting a mifepristone-induced adrenal hyperactivity. One week after adding ketoconazole to mifepristone, there was almost a 50% decrease in these values, reflecting the ability of ketoconazole to block adrenal cortisol synthesis. *we calculated the mean daily serum cortisol values (individual values were measured at 8 AM, 3 PM, and 11 PM).*

We interpreted this phenomenon as a mifepristone-induced hypercortisolism overwhelming the cortisol-inactivating capacity of the 11β-hydroxysteroid dehydrogenase type 2 (11β-HSD2); this enzyme—located in the distal tubule of the nephron—converts active cortisol into inactive cortisone, thus preventing cortisol-induced activation of the local mineralocorticoid receptor. Mifepristone blocks the glucocorticoid receptor, but not the mineralocorticoid receptor. So, excess cortisol stimulates the mineralocorticoid receptor of the distal kidney tubule, provoking excess renal sodium reabsorption and excess urinary potassium excretion.

3.2 Mifepristone (600 mg/day) plus ketoconazole (800 mg/day) combination therapy (a single week)

As predicted, the addition of ketoconazole (an antifungal agent capable of inhibiting cortisol synthesis) enhanced the anti-glucocorticoid effect of mifepristone, as reflected by a further reduction of the serum levels of triglycerides and fasting insulin and glucose levels (**Table 3**). These effects paralleled a drop of mean daily total serum cortisol and urinary free cortisol excretion, as shown in **Table 2. Table 4** shows a striking reduction of serum insulin values observed during an oral glucose tolerance test (OGTT) performed with 75 g of glucose on the last day of the combined administration, compared with the values observed 2 years earlier.

Days (Starting from Week 10)	Serum fasting triglycerides (mg/dL)	Fasting glycemia (mg/dL)	Fasting insulinemia (mU/L)
Day 1	380	180	12.0
Day 2	375	145	17.5
Day 3	300	122	13.0
Day 4	250	121	13.5
Day 5	240	135	13.6
Day 6	220	129	7.5
Day 7	230	138	7.0

Table 3.
Assessment of metabolic parameters during mifepristone (600 mg/day) plus ketoconazole (800 mg/day) combination therapy. The addition of ketoconazole to mifepristone for 7 days notoriously reduced serum fasting levels of triglycerides, glucose, and insulin to near-normal values.

Minutes	0'	30'	60'	90'	120'
Basal (1986)	61	193	357	153	>300
Combined Anti-glucocorticoid Administration (1988)	11	19	27	24	23

Table 4.
Serum insulin levels (mU/L) measured during oral glucose tolerance tests (OGTT) performed (with 75 g of glucose) at baseline (1986) and during the mifepristone plus ketoconazole combination therapy (1988). Serum insulin levels observed during the OGTT performed at the end of the combined anti-glucocorticoid administration (1988) were strikingly reduced, as compared with values observed during the baseline OGTT (performed in 1986).

Weeks	Serum fasting triglycerides (mg/dL)	Fasting glycemia (mg/dL)	Fasting insulinemia (mU/L)
11	360	160	n/a
12	438	200	n/a

Table 5.
Assessment of metabolic parameters during the second course of mifepristone therapy alone (600 mg/day). There was a substantial increase in fasting triglyceride and glucose levels after the discontinuation of ketoconazole for 7 days. Abbreviations: n/a, not available.

3.3 Second course of mifepristone therapy alone, 600 mg/day (2 weeks)

We observed a progressive deterioration of serum triglyceride and glucose values after stopping ketoconazole (**Table 5**). Unfortunately, we did not measure cortisol values during this period.

3.4 Summary of metabolic changes observed during the anti-glucocorticoid intervention

As observed in **Table 1**, mifepristone therapy alone took 2 weeks to substantially reduce serum fasting triglyceride and insulin levels, while serum fasting glucose was unchanged during this phase of anti-glucocorticoid intervention. The 1-week addition of ketoconazole produced a further reduction of serum triglycerides and a rapid drop of serum fasting glucose values (**Table 3**). However, over the next 2 weeks of the trial with mifepristone therapy alone, we observed a clear rise in serum triglyceride and glucose values (**Table 5**).

3.5 The decision to perform total (bilateral) adrenalectomy and its results

None of the observations that we made during our protocol execution negated our working hypothesis. Regarding definitive therapy for lipoatrophic diabetes, mifepristone administration was ruled out for its limited availability and expected complications. By contrast, bilateral adrenalectomy, along with a limited cortisol replacement therapy, would reduce fat exposure to high, lipolysis-inducing cortisol levels. The family and the patient agreed to the surgical procedure. After surgery, we administered a reduced but safe amount of hydrocortisone (15 mg/day, divided into daily doses: 10 mg at 8 AM and 5 mg at 3 PM). In addition, we administered fludrocortisone 0.1 mg daily to avoid excessive urinary sodium loss.

Minutes	0’	30’	60’	90’	120’
Serum glucose (mg/dL)	98	140	148	195	210
Serum insulin (mU/L)	10	45	53	47	52

Table 6.
Serum glucose and insulin values during the oral glucose tolerance test (OGTT) performed (with 75 g of glucose) 13 days following bilateral adrenalectomy, under hydrocortisone (15 mg/day) plus fludrocortisone (0.1 mg/day) replacement therapy. Serum glucose values were within the lowest diabetic range, while hyperinsulinemia was absent.

At the time of adrenalectomy, surgeons were surprised to observe a fat-devoid mesentery (**Figure 1**). The patient recovered uneventfully from the surgical procedure. After adrenalectomy, we measured fasting glucose levels daily, and we performed an OGTT (with 75 g of glucose) 2 weeks later (**Table 6**).

751

SUCCESSFUL REYERSAL OF THE INSULIN RESISTANCE OF CONGENITAL LIPOATROPHIC DIABETES (CLD) BY ANTIGLUCOCORTICOID (AGC) THERAPY (RU 486).

P. Contreras, H. Michelsen*, J. Pérez*, I. Mella* and M. Ríos*

Endocrine Section, Hospital Clínico Universidad de Chile, Santiago, **CHILE**.

Resistance to the **antilipolytic** effect of **insulin** (IN) may mediate the hyperlipidemia (type Y) of CLD. Since **glucocorticoids**, aside from their diabetogenic actions, increase **lipolylisis** we reasoned that **AGC Rx** with RU 486 might normalize hypertriglyceridemia and hyperglycemia of CLD. **RU 486** (up to 600 mg daily) was given to a 18-yr old woman with CLD. On the ninth week of treatment **Ketoconazole** (KCZ) , a steroidogenesis blocker with peripheral AGC activity was added (800 mg daily) for one week. Oral glucose tolerance tests (OGTTs) were performed in 1986 (no Rx) and again at the end of the combined therapy (1988). After KCZ was discontinued, RU Rx was maintained. Serum triglycerides (TG), fasting glycemias (G) and serum IN were measured periodically.

RESULTS	**TG**	**G**	**IN**	µUI/ml during OGTT (75 g)	
	mg/dL		**Time**	**1986**	**1988**
Basal	7,400	225	0'	61	11
RU, 4 wks	1,090	276	30'	193	19
RU, 8 "	617	227	60'	357	27
RU + KCZ	225	143	90'	153	24
RU, 10 wks	360	160	120'	>350	23
RU, 11 "	438	200			

Clinically, RU Rx induced an almost complete regression of both eruptive xanthomas and acanthosis nigricans as well as a significant weight gain (7k) and an important reduction of her hepatosplenomegaly. **Compensatory overactivity** of the **adrenal axis** brought about by RU Rx (as evidenced by urinary 17-OHCS of 45-66 mg/24 h) lead to slight **arterial hypertension** (160/100) as well as **hypokalemia** (3.4 mEq/L) and **hyperkaliuria** (56 mEq/24 h).

CONCLUSIONS : normalization of serum TG during the trial suggests that RU 486 Rx may restrain lipolysis in CLD; the IN data would indicate on the other hand that such therapy partially reverted IN resistance regarding glucose metabolization in this patient. The beneficial effects of adding KCZ to RU Rx suggests that the working hypothesis was basically correct.

Supported in part by Project M 1869 8855, Universidad de Chile

Figure 2.
The facsimile of our abstract, as it was published in the proceedings of the Endocrine Society Seventy-First Annual Meeting; June 21–24, 1989, Seattle, Washington (USA).

Twenty-four hours after the adrenalectomy, fasting serum glucose was within the normal range, followed by occasional minimal increments above the normal range in the next 2 weeks. The OGTT results showed a fasting glucose level within the normal range and a 2-h glucose level in the low diabetic range. The insulin values during the OGTT were within the normal range, although with an unusual trajectory (**Table 6**).

We performed successful adrenalectomy in our lipoatrophic patient 14 years before the adrenalectomy success observed in transgenic A-ZIP/F1 lipoatrophic mice [12].

3.6 Patient discharge and follow-up

We discharged the patient from the hospital (1988) medicated with hydrocortisone (10 mg at 8 AM and 5 mg at 3 PM) plus fludrocortisone (0.1 mg at 8 AM). We instructed her to double the fludrocortisone dose in the summer. Subsequently, she opted to be taken care of by the National Health Service (NHS) due to financial reasons. We never had the opportunity to discuss the case with her new attending diabetologists.

Likely, the idea of using a reduced but safe amount of oral hydrocortisone in this patient did not appeal to her new attending physicians. Besides, the NHS in Chile did not provide fludrocortisone at that time, so the patient likely overdosed with hydrocortisone. Despite these shortcomings, the patient got pregnant twice, having a spontaneous abortion in 2002. In 2003, aged 34, she got pregnant again and delivered a premature, 28-week baby. Her attending obstetricians reviewed the literature and discovered a single case with successful pregnancy in women with CGL [22]. They described the difficult pregnancy in a local obstetrics journal [23]. Even though triglyceride levels remained elevated (below 2000 mg/dL), these levels were substantially lower compared with those observed when we first met her (7100 mg/dL). However, the obstetrics report mentioned one episode of acute pancreatitis antedating her second pregnancy.

We presented our experience in 1989 at The Endocrine Society Meeting in Seattle [24] (**Figure 2**). However, at that time, we could not write up a paper reporting our findings simply because we could not offer a rational explanation for them.

4. Discussion

To reinterpret the therapeutic findings in this teenager, we must briefly revise crucial new knowledge accumulated in the decades since we treated her.

4.1 Extreme adipose tissue insulin resistance (Adipo-IR) at the core of CGL?

Insulin action on the adipocyte stimulates adipogenesis and lipogenesis while inhibiting lipolysis. Extreme insulin resistance in the adipose tissue (Adipo-IR) should severely reduce adipogenesis and lipogenesis. At the same time, Adipo-IR should increase lipolysis, leading to an "empty adipocyte" syndrome. It is conceivable that glucocorticoid action on the adipocyte somehow mediates Adipo-IR. Once the adipocyte becomes triglyceride-depleted, leptin secretion should severely fall, resulting in hypoleptinemia. The latter may lead to adrenal hyperactivity (as seen in murine models of CGL), resulting in hypercorticosteronemia [12]. In patients with CGL, the hypothetical high circulating free cortisol levels (elevated serum total cortisol levels plus hyperinsulinemia-induced low transcortin levels) would perpetuate the increased lipolysis.

Adipo-IR is present at both extremes of adipocyte's triglyceride storage: triglyceride-replete adipocytes and empty adipocytes (as seen in obesity and CGL, respectively). In both cases, ectopic triglyceride storage in lean organs (liver, muscle, pancreatic beta cell, and skin) replaces further adipocyte triglyceride storage. Lipotoxicity in the liver increases the hepatic glucose output. Lipotoxicity in muscles reduces their insulin-mediated glucose uptake. Finally, beta-cell lipotoxicity induces cell apoptosis. The degree of lean tissue lipotoxicity is severe in CGL patients with "empty adipocytes." By contrast, in obese subjects, lipotoxicity is considerably lighter (triglyceride-replete adipocytes). If mifepristone administration ameliorates Adipo-IR, it is logical to expect a metabolic improvement of both CGL and obesity.

4.2 Mifepristone and adipose tissue insulin sensitivity

We know that mifepristone improves glucose tolerance and insulin sensitivity in patients with Cushing's syndrome [25]. However, the specific effect of the drug on adipose tissue's insulin sensitivity had remained unexplored. In 2021, an NIH group reported that mifepristone improves adipose tissue insulin sensitivity in insulin-resistant individuals [26]. Sixteen overweight or obese subjects with prediabetes or mild type 2 diabetes (without Cushing's syndrome) received either mifepristone (200 mg/day; 50 mg 4 times a day) or placebo for 9 days with a washout period of 8 weeks. At baseline and following mifepristone and placebo administration, the subjects had a 75-g OGTT and a frequently sampled intravenous glucose tolerance test (FSIVGTT). Whole-body insulin sensitivity was estimated on these subjects calculating three indices: Insulin Sensitivity Index (SI), Matsuda index (MI), and Oral Glucose Insulin Sensitivity Index (OGIS). These indices were not modified by mifepristone 200 mg daily. However, there were significant improvements in the adipose tissue insulin resistance index (Adipo-IR index) (a surrogate marker of fasting adipose-tissue insulin resistance, calculated as the product of fasting insulin and fasting free fatty acids) and in the adipose tissue insulin sensitivity index (Adipo-S_I index, defined as the ratio of the slope of the linear decrease in natural log transformed free fatty acids during the first 90 minutes of the FSIVGTT and the area under the curve of serum insulin during that 90-minute period) [26]. In addition, mifepristone increased insulin clearance but did not modify either insulin secretion or beta-cell glucose sensitivity. Mifepristone use reduced fasting serum glucose, insulin, and triglycerides. Also, the areas under the curve of daily serum ACTH and cortisol values were significantly higher during mifepristone administration. Urinary free cortisol values also rose significantly. Thus, mifepristone 200 mg/day (divided into four 50-mg daily doses) administered to 16 insulin-resistant subjects reproduced our findings using 600 mg daily (divided into three 200 mg doses): serum and urinary cortisol values rose, while serum glucose, insulin, and triglyceride values fell.

Therefore, mifepristone (600 mg/day) should have improved the adipose tissue insulin sensitivity in our patient. Since we did not measure serum FFAs, we cannot evaluate the Adipo-IR index in our patient. However, using a raw estimation of adipose tissue's insulin resistance—the product of insulin (mU/L) times fasting triglycerides (mg/dL), we obtain the following results: mifepristone alone: at baseline, >2,960,000; 9th week, 4936; mifepristone plus ketoconazole combination therapy: first day, 4560; 7th day, 1610. As a reference, a person with a fasting serum insulin value of 13 mU/mL and 150 mg/dL of fasting triglycerides would have a calculated value of 1950 for this parameter. Therefore, this raw estimation of the adipose tissue's insulin resistance shows a strikingly positive effect of mifepristone, which is further reinforced by the addition of ketoconazole (>99.9% reduction).

A recent Chinese study on the Adipo-IR index and metabolic syndrome [27] reported mean data from six groups of subjects (three groups for each sex) on insulin and triglyceride values. These data allowed us the calculation of our raw adipose tissue insulin resistance index in 20 control females (612.4), 26 obese women without metabolic syndrome (1165.0), and 85 obese women with metabolic syndrome (3017.9). There was a strong, positive correlation of 0.958 between their published averaged Adipo-IR indices and their corresponding calculated raw Adipo-IR indices.

So, this proposed raw estimation of adipose tissue insulin resistance should be helpful in the clinical setting. Both a serum fasting triglyceride value >130 mg/dL and a serum fasting insulin value >13.2 mU/L suggest the presence of insulin resistance. Therefore, a value above 1716 (13.2 times 130) for this raw index would strongly indicate the presence of adipose tissue insulin resistance. Likely, values for this surrogate index in non-insulin-resistant individuals should be less than 1000 (corresponding to a serum insulin value around 7.5 mU/L and a serum triglyceride value around 130 mg/dL).

4.3 Adrenalectomy and insulin resistance

When we received this patient, we knew that patients with Addison's disease were lean, insulin-sensitive, and prone to hypoglycemia. On the contrary, patients with Cushing's syndrome are obese, insulin-resistant, and prone to hyperglycemia. Glucocorticoids promote both obesity and insulin resistance, thus deteriorating diabetes control. By contrast, adrenalectomy benefits diabetes control in patients with Cushing's syndrome. Of course, we did not know in 1988 that adrenalectomy would improve diabetes in A-ZIP/F1 lipoatrophic mice [12]. Adrenalectomy in this murine model of CGL ameliorates liver and muscle insulin sensitivity. The fact that mice lacking leptin synthesis or leptin action (*ob/ob* and db/db mice, respectively) are both obese and insulin-resistant [28] suggests that leptin action somehow protects them from insulin resistance. The beneficial effects of adrenalectomy in rodents lacking leptin action [29] indicate that the adrenal gland is necessary for these mice to develop insulin resistance. In summary, we need to find the intermediate steps between insufficient leptin action and insulin resistance. In experimental animals with hypoleptinemia, the adrenal gland appears to mediate the development of insulin resistance.

4.4 The new knowledge on Berardinelli-Seip syndrome and its relationship with leptin

The clinical and metabolic improvements observed in our patient during the anti-glucocorticoid intervention were beyond our expectations. The significant weight gain of our patient is encouraging and particularly intriguing. It suggests *de novo* storage of triglycerides in the patient's fat depots. If this latter supposition is true, then one wonders whether the supposedly much-reduced leptin and adiponectin levels at baseline rose when fat progressively accumulated within the adipocytes during anti-glucocorticoid therapy. Future research will probably answer these intriguing questions. Although we realized that the anti-glucocorticoid therapy notoriously improved the abnormal adipocyte physiology of our patient, we did not disclose the mechanism(s) involved. In any case, the beneficial effects of the anti-glucocorticoid treatment support the notion of a detrimental action of endogenous cortisol on the adipocyte physiology in this CGL patient.

Now, we can attempt to offer a rational explanation concerning the effects of mifepristone in our patient with Berardinelli-Seip Syndrome. Nowadays, we know several key pieces of crucial importance, such as the discovery of leptin and its functions [9]. A key concept is that leptin exerts an inhibitory effect on the hypothalamic–pituitary–adrenal axis [30]. Moreover, the loss of leptin-induced inhibition of the hypothalamic–pituitary–adrenal axis provokes gross metabolic dysfunctions. For instance, hepatic gluconeogenesis is largely augmented in murine models of poorly controlled type 1 diabetes, having severely low insulin levels [31]. Shortly after leptin discovery, it was evident that CGL patients exhibited severe hypoleptinemia [32]. In 1998, the new era of transgenic mice with lipoatrophic diabetes introduced revolutionary concepts in the field [7, 8]. The less fat-deficient mice responded well to leptin treatment, whereas the severely fat-devoid A-ZIP/F1 mice responded poorly. These mice exhibit hypercorticosteronemia, indicating an overactivity of their adrenal axes. Intravenous leptin infusions reduce adrenal gland overactivity in these mice. When these A-ZIP/F1 mice were adrenalectomized to abate their hypercorticosteronemia, they experienced significant increments in peripheral and hepatic insulin sensitivity [12]. Again, another piece of evidence is that an adrenal gland is necessary for these leptin-deficient mice to develop diabetes.

Patients with CGL treated with recombinant leptin usually respond well to the hormone [4]. To our knowledge, nobody has yet reported that patients with CGL have an overactive adrenal axis, in parallel with the findings observed in murine models of CGL. Unfortunately, it did not occur to us to evaluate the hypothalamic–pituitary–adrenal axis before the trial began. On the other hand, transcortin (also known as CBG or corticosteroid-binding globulin; the protein produced in the liver that transports cortisol in the blood) expression is reduced by hyperinsulinemia [33]. Patients with CGL should theoretically exhibit high levels of serum free cortisol secondary to both hypoleptinemia-induced adrenal gland overactivity and low transcortin levels (due to hyperinsulinemia-induced reduction in hepatic secretion of transcortin).

If leptin deficiency in humans indeed results in the lack of leptin-mediated inhibition of the hypothalamic–pituitary–adrenal axis, a logical consequence of this hormonal deficiency would be the overactivity of the adrenal glands. This situation would be revealed either by high serum total or free cortisol levels, paralleling the hypercorticosteronemia of leptin-deficient rodents. Lipolysis in insulin-resistant subjects should increase due to resistance to insulin-induced HSL inhibition. If the adrenal axis becomes overactive, the permissive role of cortisol on HSL activation should increase. A foreseeable result of this phenomenon is an enhanced lipolysis. The high efflux of FFAs and glycerol in the blood will increase hepatic gluconeogenesis, thus impairing glucose homeostasis. Under this situation, triglycerides would migrate from the adipocytes (normotopic storage) into lean organs (ectopic storage). Fat relocation should produce a "triglyceride-depleted adipocyte." On the other hand, fat relocation and ectopic fat accumulation should reduce leptin secretion and induce lipotoxicity in lean organs such as the liver, skeletal muscles, and endocrine pancreas.

5. Conclusions

a) If hypoleptinemia drives adrenal axis hyperactivity in CGL (**Figure 3**), three interventions (recombinant leptin, anti-glucocorticoids, and bilateral adrenalectomy) should reduce fat exposure to cortisol action in CGL patients (**Figure 4**). Moreover, on the horizon, the nonpeptide, oral ACTH antagonist CRN04894 [34] might become a promising therapeutic alternative. If ACTH antagonists reach the market and prove safe for chronic use, administration of these drugs in CGL patients may be beneficial due to their adrenal-blocking properties.

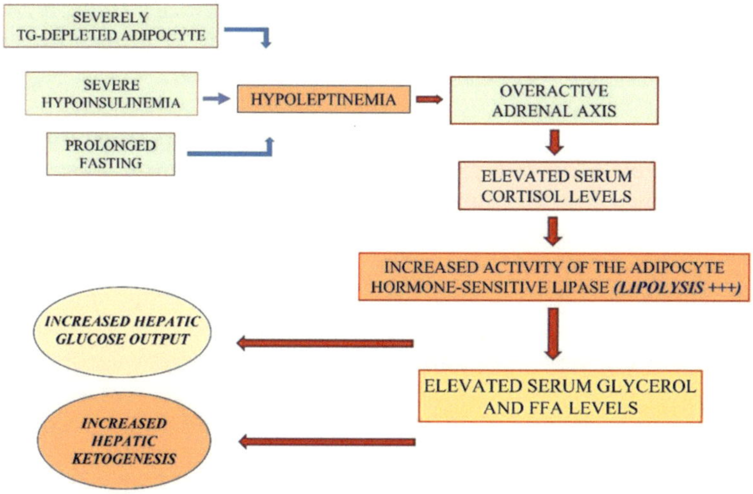

Figure 3.
Potential pathophysiological mechanisms underlying the hypoleptinemia-induced hyperactivity of the hypothalamic–pituitary–adrenal axis (adrenal axis, for short) and subsequent unrestrained adipose tissue lipolysis. Since leptin restrains the hypothalamic–pituitary–adrenal axis, any cause of severe hypoleptinemia (CGL, severe hypoinsulinemia of diabetic ketoacidosis, and prolonged fasting) should result in an overactive adrenal axis. Fat exposure to excess serum cortisol should stimulate adipocyte hormone-sensitive lipase (HSL) and increase lipolysis. Abbreviations: FFA, free fatty acids; TG, triglycerides.

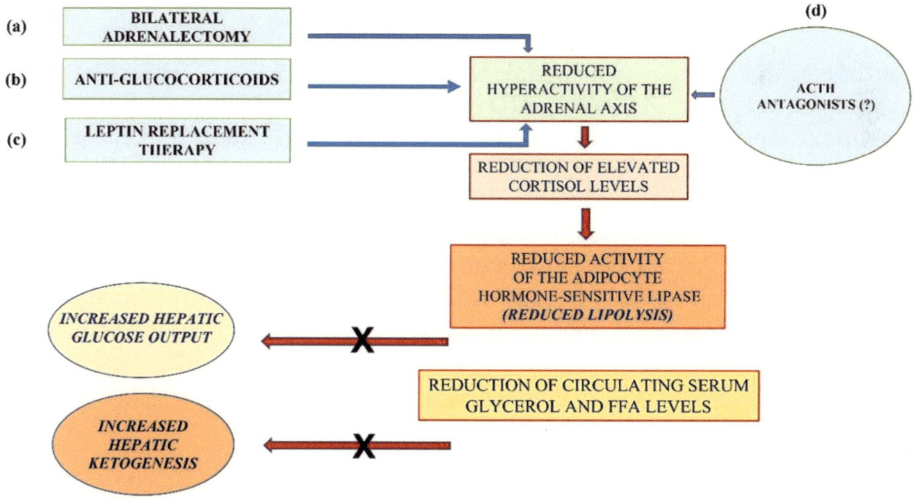

Figure 4.
Predicted therapeutic interventions aimed at reducing fat exposure to excessive cortisol levels in patients with Berardinelli-Seip syndrome (congenital generalized lipodystrophy). According to our hypothesis, adrenalectomy (a), anti-glucocorticoid therapy (b), and leptin replacement (c) should result in a restrained activity of the hypothalamic–pituitary–adrenal axis (adrenal axis, for short), reducing fat depots exposure to free cortisol levels. The same effects should result from using future ACTH antagonists (d). Consequently, any of these four interventions should diminish the degree of lipolysis. In turn, reduced lipolysis should ameliorate ectopic fat storage in lean organs (liver, muscle, pancreatic beta cells, and skin), improving tissue insulin sensitivity. Abbreviation: ACTH, adrenocorticotropic hormone; FFA, free fatty acids.

b) Mifepristone is not suitable for patients with CGL, since it induces adrenal axis overactivity. This fact anticipates complications such as adrenal hyperplasia and hypercortisolemia-induced hypermineralocortisolism.

c) Bilateral, total adrenalectomy might become a feasible therapeutic alternative for CGL patients. Currently, laparoscopic adrenalectomy entails a low long-term risk to patients. Adrenalectomized patients are perfectly able to manage their hormone replacement therapy.

d) The exact mechanism by which anti-glucocorticoid therapy resulted in the notable metabolic improvement observed in our patient remains unknown and should be investigated. Simultaneous defects in adipogenesis, lipogenesis, and lipolysis may cause lipodystrophy in patients with CGL. "Runaway lipolysis" by itself as the single culprit of lipodystrophy remains an unproven possibility.

e) The storage of fat in adipose tissue depends on the correct functioning of adipogenesis, lipogenesis, and lipolysis, working as a whole process. It may be plausible that a failure in just one of these three elements is sufficient to derange the whole process, leading to lipodystrophy.

f) An urgent task is to study the status of the adrenal axis in patients with untreated CGL. If this axis turns out to be overactive, future clinical trials with anti-glucocorticoids in patients with CGL are warranted.

Acknowledgements

This author is indebted to several people that facilitated this work. In the first place, thanks are due to Harold Michelsen, MD (deceased), who asked me to develop a therapeutic strategy for this complex patient after the lack of success of the usual medicines to treat her diabetes and dyslipidemia. This author is also grateful to the endocrinology colleagues in our Unit, who were brave enough to endorse our proposed—unheard-of—strategy to attempt a rational treatment of our patient. This author is also grateful to our patient and her family, who trusted our Unit in times of therapeutical uncertainty. They not only accepted the anti-glucocorticoid therapeutic approach but also dared to try bilateral, irreversible adrenalectomy after our metabolic success. Lastly, but not least, this author must thank Inés Vega, RN, and her crew for helping the patient along the road to achieving better health.

Conflicts of interest

The author declares no conflict of interest.

Author details

Patricio H. Contreras
Fundación Médica San Cristóbal, Santiago, Chile

*Address all correspondence to: pathomero@gmail.com

References

[1] Mantzoros CS. Lipodystrophic syndromes. Uptodate. Topic updated 8th June 2021

[2] Tsoukas MA, Mantzoros CS. Lipodystrophy syndromes. Chapter 37. In: Jameson JL, DeGroot LJ, editors. Endocrinology: Adult and Pediatric. 7th ed. Elsevier;2016. pp. 648-661e5

[3] de Azevedo Medeiros LB, Candido Dantas VK, Craveiro Sarmento AS, Agnes-Lima LF, Meireles AL, Xavier Nobre TT, et al. High prevalence of Berardinelli-Seip congenital lipodystrophy in Rio Grande do Norte state, Northeast Brazil. Diabetology and Metabolic Syndrome. 2017;**9**(1):80-86. DOI: 10.1186/s13098-017-0280-7

[4] Oral EA, Simha V, Ruiz E, Andewelt A, Premkumar A, Snell P, et al. Leptin replacement therapy for lipodystrophy. The New England Journal of Medicine. 2002;**346**(8):570-578. DOI: 10.1056/NEJMoa012437

[5] Berardinelli W. An undiagnosed endocrinometabolic syndrome: Report of 2 cases. The Journal of Clinical Endocrinology and Metabolism. 1954;**14**(2):193-204. DOI: 10.1210/jcem-14-2-193

[6] Seip M. Lipodystrophy and gigantism with associated endocrine manifestations. A new diencephalic syndrome? Acta Paediatrica. 1959;**48**:555-574

[7] Moitra J, Mason MM, Olive M, Krylov D, Gavrilova O, Marcus-Samuels B, et al. Life without white fat: A transgenic mouse. Genes & Development. 1998;**12**:3168-3181. DOI: 10.1101/gad.12.20.3168

[8] Shimomura I, Hammer RE, Richardson JA, Ikemoto S, Bashmakov Y, Goldstein JL, et al. Insulin resistance and diabetes mellitus in transgenic mice expressing nuclear SREBP-1c in adipose tissue: Model for congenital generalized lipodystrophy. Genes & Development. 1998;**12**:3182-3194. DOI: 10.1101/gad.12.20.3182

[9] Zhang Y, Proenca R, Maffei M, Barone M, Leopold L, Friedman JM. Positional cloning of the mouse *obese* gene and its human homologue. Nature. 1994;**372**:425-432. DOI: 10.1038/372425a0

[10] Shimomura I, Hammer RE, Ikemoto S, Brown MS, Goldstein JL. Leptin reverses insulin resistance and diabetes mellitus in mice with congenital lipodystrophy. Nature. 1999;**401**(6748):73-76. DOI: 10.1038/43448

[11] Reitman ML, Gavrilova O. A-ZIP/F-1 mice lacking white fat: A model for understanding lipoatrophic diabetes. International Journal of Obesity and Related Metabolic Disorders. 2000; **24**(Suppl 4):S11-S14. DOI: 10.1038/sj.ijo.0801493

[12] Haluzik M, Dietz KR, Kim JK, Marcus-Samuels B, Shulman GI, Gavrilova O, et al. Adrenalectomy improves diabetes in A-ZIP/F-1 lipoatrophic mice by increasing both liver and muscle insulin sensitivity. Diabetes. 2002;**51**:2113-2118. DOI: 10.2337/diabetes.51.7.2113

[13] FDA Approves Myalept. 2014. Available from: https://www.drugs.com/newdrugs/fda-approves-myalept-generalized-lipodystrophy-4010.html [Accessed: December 13, 2021]

[14] Cortés VA, David E. Curtis DE, Sukumaran S, Shao X, Parameswara V, Rashid S, et al. Molecular mechanisms of hepatic steatosis and insulin resistance

in the AGPAT2-deficient mouse model of congenital generalized lipodystrophy. Cell Metabolism. 2009;**9**:165-176. DOI: 10.1016/j.cmet.2009.01.002

[15] Cui X, Wang Y, Tang Y, Liu Y, Zhao L, Deng J, et al. Seipin ablation in mice results in severe generalized lipodystrophy. Human Molecular Genetics. 2011;**20**:3022-3030. DOI: 10.1093/hmg/ddr205

[16] Chen W, Chang B, Saha P, Hartig SM, Li L, Reddy VT, et al. Berardinelli-Seip congenital lipodystrophy 2/Seipin is a cell-autonomous regulator of lipolysis essential for adipocyte differentiation. Molecular and Cellular Biology. 2012;**32**(6):1099-1111. DOI: 10.1128/MCB.06465-11

[17] Rao MJ, Goodman JM. Seipin: Harvesting fat and keeping adipocytes healthy. Trends in Cell Biology. 2021;**11**:912-923. DOI: 10.1016/j.tcb.2021.06.003

[18] Cautivo KM, Lizama CO, Tapia PJ, Agarwal AK, Garg A, Horton JD, et al. AGPAT2 is essential for postnatal development and maintenance of white and brown adipose tissue. Molecular Metabolism. 2016;**5**:491-505. DOI: 10.1016/j.molmet.2016.05.004

[19] Tansey JT, Sztalryd C, Gruia-Gray J, Roush DL, Zee JV, Gavrilova O, et al. Perilipin ablation results in a lean mouse with aberrant adipocyte lipolysis, enhanced leptin production, and resistance to diet-induced obesity. Proceedings of the National Academy of Sciences of the United States of America. 2001;**98**(11):6494-6499. DOI: 10.1073/pnas.101042998

[20] Contreras P, Altieri E, Liberman C, Gac A, Rojas A, Ibarra A, et al. Adrenal rest tumor of the liver causing Cushing's syndrome: Treatment with ketoconazole preceding an apparent surgical cure. The Journal of Clinical Endocrinology and Metabolism. 1985;**60**(1):21-28. DOI: 10.1210/jcem-60-1-21

[21] Contreras P, Rojas A, Biagini L, González P, Massardo T. Regression of metastatic adrenal carcinoma during palliative ketoconazole treatment. Lancet. 1985;**2**:151-152. DOI: 10.1016/s0140-6736(85)90251-x

[22] Taylor SI, Arioglu E. Syndromes associated with insulin resistance and acanthosis nigricans. Journal of Basic and Clinical Physiology and Pharmacology. 1998;**9**(2-4):419-439. DOI: 10.1515/jbcpp.1998.9.2-4.419

[23] Orellana R, Bustos JC, Rojas N, Godoy M, Ramírez J. Éxito reproductivo en embarazo de madre portadora de diabetes lipoatrófica generalizada. Revista Chilena de Obstetricia y Ginecología. 2004;**69**(3):242-245. DOI: 10.4067/S0717-75262004000300011

[24] Contreras P, Michelsen H, Pérez J, Ríos M. Successful reversal of the insulin resistance of congenital lipoatrophic diabetes (CLD) by antiglucocorticoid (AGC) therapy (RU 486). Abstract 751. In: The Endocrine Society Seventy-First Annual Meeting. Washington, USA: Seattle; 21-24 June 1989

[25] Wallia A, Colleran K, Purnell JQ, Molitch ME. Improvement in insulin sensitivity during mifepristone treatment of Cushing syndrome: Early and late effects. Diabetes Care. 2013;**36**(9):e147-e148. DOI: 10.2337/dc13-0246

[26] Gubbi S, Muniyappa R, Sharma ST, Grewal S, McGlotten R, Nieman LK. Mifepristone improves adipose tissue insulin sensitivity in insulin resistant individuals. The Journal of Clinical Endocrinology and Metabolism.

2021;**106**(5):1501-1515. DOI: 10.1210/clinem/dgab046

[27] Zhang K, Pan H, Wang L, Yang H, Zhu H, Gong F. Adipose tissue insulin resistance is closely associated with metabolic syndrome in northern Chinese populations. Diabetes, Metabolic Syndrome and Obesity: Targets and Therapy. 2021;**14**:1117-1128. DOI: 10.2147/DMSO.S291350

[28] Wang B, Chandrasekera PC, Pippin J. Leptin- and leptin receptor-deficient rodent models: Relevance for human type 2 diabetes. Current Diabetes Reviews. 2014;**10**(2):131-145. DOI: 10.2174/1573399810666140508121012

[29] Makimura H, Mizuno TM, Roberts J, Silverstein J, Beasley J, Mobbs CV. Adrenalectomy reverses obese phenotype and restores hypothalamic melanocortin tone in leptin-deficient Ob/Ob mice. Diabetes. 2000;**49**(11):1917-1923. DOI: 10.2337/diabetes.49.11.1917

[30] Perry RJ, Zhang XM, Zhang D, Kumashiro N, Camporez JPG, Cline GW, et al. Leptin reverses diabetes by suppression of the hypothalamic-pituitary-adrenal axis. Nature Medicine. 2014;**20**(7):759-763. DOI: 10.1038/nm.3579

[31] Perry RJ, Peng L, Abulizi A, Kennedy L, Cline GW, Shulman GI. Mechanism for leptin's acute insulin-independent effect to reverse diabetic ketoacidosis. The Journal of Clinical Investigation. 2017;**127**(2):657-669. DOI: 10.1172/JCI88477

[32] Haque WA, Shimomura I, Matsuzawa Y, Garg A. Serum adiponectin and leptin levels in patients with lipodystrophies. The Journal of Clinical Endocrinology and Metabolism. 2002;**87**:2395-2398. DOI: 10.1210/jcem.87.5.8624

[33] Fernández-Real JM, Grasa M, Casamitjana R, Pugeat M, Barret C, Ricart W. Plasma total and glycosylated corticosteroid-binding globulin levels are associated with insulin secretion. The Journal of Clinical Endocrinology and Metabolism. 1999;**84**:3192-3196. DOI: 10.1210/jcem.84.9.5946

[34] Fowler MA, Kusnetzow AK, Han S, Reinhart R, Kim SH, et al. Effects of CRN04894, a nonpeptide orally bioavailable ACTH antagonist, on corticosterone in rodent models of ACTH excess. Endocrine Society's annual ENDO 2021 Oral Sessions. Available from: https://crinetics.com/wp-content/uploads/2021/03/Melissa_Effects-of-CRN04894-a-Nonpeptide-Orally-Bioavailable-ACTH-Antagonist-on-Corticosterone-in-Rodent-Models-of-ACTH-Excess.pdf [Accessed: December 13, 2021]